I0145946

SANDRA KELLY

THE DRAGONS OF DECAGON

A DRAGON'S TALE

The Dragons of Decagon
Copyright © 2022 by Sandra Kelly. All rights reserved.

All rights reserved. No part of this book may be reproduced or transmitted in any form or by any means, electronic or mechanical, including photocopying, recording, or by any information storage and retrieval system without express written permission from the author, except in the case of brief quotations embodied in critical reviews and certain other noncommercial uses permitted by copyright law.

Published in the United States of America

Brilliant Books Literary
137 Forest Park Lane Thomasville
North Carolina 27360 USA

A Dragons Tale

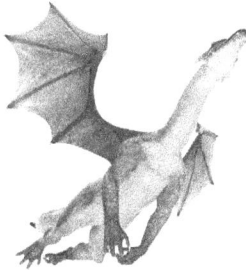

ONCE long ago, on a distant mountain called Decagon, life was very different from what we humans know now. This mountain had ten huge sides. Each side had forests, large valleys, rivers and lakes. Each mountainside was beautiful in its own way, all different but all beautiful, except one side. It was grey and murky and was always referred to as The Dark Side. Not much was known about the place, except it had a massive castle on it and was guarded by fearsome beasts. This could be why no one ever came out of there.

Our tale begins with a little creature called Green by her keepers; I believe you would call them ogres.

Green was about four feet high and spent most of her life in a cage, and she had never known anything else except when she was sent on a job. Green was used as a messenger because she could fly. Also, she had leathery scaly skin, making it possible to fly in all weather. Her messages were kept dry in a sort of pocket flap under the scales on her chest. It may sound exciting to use, but Green was a prisoner. When she left with a message, she always knew that the grawk would follow her like a guard dog and kill her if she tried to escape. So, she always returned, not that she had anywhere else to go.

Grawks were nasty, big, birdlike creatures, a sort of cross between a gryphon and a large hawk.

They were not very clever, but they obeyed every order given to them by the ogres. They always eyed Green up like a tasty snack, but I digress. Our tale is not always a nice one because of the horrible things that can happen, so be warned.

HOW THE DRAGONS FOUND EACH OTHER AND BECAME THE DRAGONS OF DECAGON

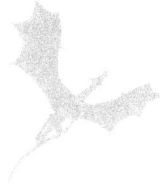

CHAPTER

1

Green had been tasked by her ogre masters with delivering a very special message to the other side of the valley. This would take around an hour to deliver, and with any luck, Green would be back before dark. This would mean that she would be able to get something to eat as a late return could mean she'd have to go hungry, and not for the first time.

The sky started to darken on the journey, and gusts of wind blew Green off course. Even though she was being blown around, her grawk minder still screeched at Green to go the right way.

Suddenly, a storm came out of nowhere, and poor Green was battered around by the wind and the rain. Green realised that she was lost and that her minder, the grawk, had vanished. *Typical, it's gone and found shelter and left me out in this",* thought Green, who was realising that she was alone for the first time in her life. Shivering with cold, Green looked as far as she could see in the dark skies. *"Perhaps I can find shelter till this passes, and I can get my bearings again,"* she told herself.

But there was no let-up in the storm. It seemed as though whatever direction Green flew in, the storm still surrounded Green. Continuing to try and find refuge, Green thought she saw a shadow, and she headed towards it, but it vanished. *"That's funny. Maybe it is that grawk trying to find me,"* as the idea of freedom took hold, she thought, *"Stupid thing as if I'm going to let it know where I am. I can go where I want, away from here, wherever away is I can find it and .... Do what, anything must be better than being with those ogres and grawks."*

Flying on, but getting more and more tired, Green realised she had to stop soon, or she could crash and damage her wings. She was very proud of her wings; they were beautiful, with lovely green scales shimmering even in the storm's poor light. In the sunlight, they were better than ever. While she was musing over this, she caught sight of the shadow again. It was big, well larger than a grawk. Starting to feel a little bit more nervous now about what it could be. Green looked for somewhere to land and hide till the storm passed.

Spotting a rocky outcrop with trees on it, Green headed for the cover it would give from both the storm and whatever was out there. As she tried to land, a quick gust caught her and rolled her round and round until she eventually stopped under a large Gushyberry tree. These trees have delicious big fruits on them, and when you bite into them, the juice gushes into your mouth. The very thought of them made Greens' tummy rumble really loudly, and in the wind, she thought she heard a chuckle.

"Who is there?" she asked, looking around and putting her back to the tree; she saw nothing.

"Just wind, I must be getting twitchy, imagining things. Probably because I am hungry", Green muttered to herself. "I'm always hungry, and the ogres do not give me a lot of food."

To have a Gushyberry all to herself was a dream come true. She then looked up at all the fruit, and it was hers. Green fluttered her wings, rising in a slow hover; she reached some of the fruit. She was pulling it off the branches and letting it drop. She carried onto another branch to get more. "Might as well get breakfast as well while I am up here," she said. She let her hover slowly lower to the ground when about twenty lay below.

Just as she landed, out of the corner of her eye, she saw movement. Turning quickly, she saw an eye in the leaves of a bush. When she jumped back in surprise, her foot went into a gushyberry, and juice squirted everywhere. There was no doubt that giggles were coming out of the bush this time.

"Who is there?" Green asked, more annoyed than scared. "Who are you? Show yourself"?.

Slowly a head appeared, a blue head followed by a body, tail and gorgeous iridescent wings. Flabbergasted, Green just stared at this being. Bigger than her by a good six feet and longer, the creature just stood there with a cheeky grin on its face.

"Who are you?" asked Green. "And what are you?. Are you going to hurt me? I will fight you!"

Frowning, the creature moved slowly forward. "What do you mean, what am I? I'm a dragon the same as you. My name is Meteor. What's yours?"

"Green", she answered without thinking. "What do you mean I am a dragon? You are big, and I'm not."

Meteor looked at her and answered, "You're only a baby dragon; that's why you are small at the moment. You'll grow. Can we eat some of these now? I'm starving!"

Green paused, unsure whether to eat or run. In the end, her tummy gurgled this time, which set Meteor off laughing again. "Come on, I'm not going to hurt you. We dragons look after each other very carefully".

"How many are there? Green asked, picking up a gushyberry, biting carefully, and slurping the juice out before eating the delicious fruit.

Meteor just picked one up and popped it into his mouth. Then, with a blissful sigh, he squished it in his mouth. "Mmmmm, I love these. They are yummy". Picking up another, he looked at her and said, "You don't have to be frightened or alone anymore, you know. I was sent to look after you. Once Rainbow got rid of the grawk, he sent me on ahead while he scouted around, but he did help you get here with his storm power".

Green looked at him, stunned, not saying a word. Meteor picked up another fruit and gave it to her, making sure his claws didn't split the fruit."Have some more to eat. We have a ways to go tomorrow to meet up with Rainbow".

"Who or what is Rainbow?" Green asked while picking up another berry. She waited for an answer before biting into it.

"Rainbow is the finest dragon you will ever meet. He looks after us all and keeps the mountain valleys safe for us and the younglings. There are other older dragons as well, but they do the teaching, showing the younglings how to be a dragon, make fire, when to breathe fire, how to hunt and forage for food, and lots of other stuff that's cool to know. The best lesson of all is how to fly, but you have learnt that one yourself, haven't you?"

"How many dragons are there?" Green asked, unsure if she wanted to know; besides, there couldn't be that many. She had never seen one till now, and she had been flying around for a few years now.

Meteor thought for a minute and then surprised her with a question. "Do you know how the mountain got its name Decagon? It has ten sides, and each side is like a little country with woods, valleys, streams and lakes. And, each one is different. Dragons are on eight sides—about forty or fifty at a guess. Only the older ones know exactly how many. There is a valley where the younglings are raised until it is time to fly. Then they go to another valley on their first flight. It's not far, so it is easy for them. It is like going to a new class each year, and each valley you move to has more dragons of different abilities. So, you learn from them as well as the older ones. Then, when you have learnt what you need to know, you will live in Rainbows' valley with your parents and relatives'.

"Isn't it lonely not to have parents to bring you up?" asked Green. "I've always wanted to know who my parents were".

Meteor looked at her, puzzled. "You do know we hatch from Dragon eggs, don't you? All the eggs are laid in a huge nest, and everyone takes turns looking after them, turning them, singing to them, talking to them. So, until you grow up and get your final colour, you won't know who yours are. You know, blues to blues, golds to golds. It's simple, and we grow up to be independent and free to be who we want to be without elders dictating that we should be warriors, teachers, scouts, all good dragon stuff".

"I don't know anything," Green said with a sob in her voice. "I only know the cage in the ogres' place, and I didn't know who or what I was. I only found I could fly when the ogres kept me so hungry I tried to get up on the shelf where there were some berries to eat."

"Poor little Green," said Meteor, giving her a dragon hug. "You have been badly treated. Well, that ends now! You will soon be safe with all our dragons to look after you. I bet you don't even know how to play, do you?"

Just then, Meteor went still, as if he were listening to someone, then he moved into action.

"Quick, pick up the berry skins and hide them, then get into the woods a bit and hide. I'll be with you in a minute, and we've got trouble heading our way."

Green grabbed the fruit skins and threw them as far into the bushes as she could. "What's wrong? What's coming?" said Green.

But, Meteor was flapping his wings to lift the grass which had been flattened. In seconds, there was no trace that they had been there.

"Come on, we have to hide," he said.

Scared now, Green did as she was told and went back through bushes and into the woods. Soon Green was joined byMeteor, and they hid behind some big rocks and bushes.

"What is happening?" questioned Green.

"There are some goblins headed this way, too many to fight, so we use sneaky tactics, just don't make a sound. I dropped some full gushyberries on the ground, so with a bit of luck, they will stay by the tree and eat them, and the ones that burst will cover any smell of us," whispered Meteor.

"What are goblins?" whispered Green, looking and listening carefully but ready to use her claws if she needed to.

"They are a sort of little cousins of the ogres, nasty little blighters with big ziggyzaggy teeth that are pointy. They fly around on grawks. Rainbow spotted them searching the valley below at the other end. Are they searching for you?" asked Meteor.

"I don't know! Why would they? They don't even know I am alive. That storm blew me right away from the ogres, and even the grawk lost me. I must be at least two hundred miles into new territory, and I don't even know where I am!" said Green.

"Quiet", whispered Meteor, "and keep still, they are nearly here! Oh, dragon plop! There's four of them!"

Green stayed as still as possible, just using her eyes to search around them. Her left nostril twitched, then her right one and the smell got stronger slowly.

Meteor whispered, "Whichever nostril twitches first, that's the direction they are coming from. It's the stink. We hate it, so be prepared, and it will only get worse, so use your filter."

"What filter?" she asked, looking at Meteor slowly.

Meteor explained, "We have a filter so we can close our noses off. Shut your left eye in a double blink, and then you will feel it move, then the same with the right eye. Can you feel it?"

Green did as Meteor suggested and felt something move, but she could still breathe. "The smells' gone," she said wonderingly.

"It will help take the worst off so that you're not sick," said Meteor, "we usually are the first time we come across goblin stink!"

"I've smelled that before," said Green, "very faintly though. When I delivered to some ogres."

"What did you deliver?" asked Meteor.

"A written message."

"Do you know what it said?" queried Meteor

"I don't know. I can't read," answered Green.

"That's a shame," said Meteor. "It might have told us what they were up to."

"I still have the message that I didn't deliver," said Green.

Sure enough, four hideous looking and smelling creatures appeared from the bushes by the gushyberry tree. They first sniffed the air and looked all around them, but it was apparent that all they could smell was the juice of the burst ripe berries on the floor. Feeling safe, they set to and started gorging themselves with the fruit Meteor had left like windfalls on the ground. Slobbering and chomping, they ate their way through about fifty gushyberries. Some were the size of a man's head! They just carried on gobbling. I think that is how they got their name originally.

Green and Meteor were in a bit of a situation with four goblins feeding their faces under the gushyberry tree only about two hundred yards away from where our two dragons were hiding out in rocks and bushes.

Just in case there were more goblins around, Rainbow had told Meteor not to be found, and that help was on its way.

"How long do we have to wait?" asked Green.

"Who knows," answered Meteor. "I don't know who's coming, but it won't be too soon for me. I'm getting stiff here. Whoever comes will let me know they are here anyway. You might as well try and sleep. You don't snore, do you? That would give us away."

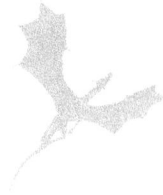

CHAPTER

2

Green curled up the best she could and dozed off, vaguely aware of a buzz in her head, like someone talking but far away. It was a comforting sound, knowing someone else was with them, even if just in her dreams.

Slowly Green woke up to become aware of Meteors claws across her mouth.

"Shh, don't move or make a sound. One of the goblins is wandering around here; I don't know what he is doing away from the others. Oh." whispered Meteor, "he is having a pee!"

Sure enough, the goblin started back out towards the gushyberry tree when he had finished. Then, he stopped and sniffed the air. Never moving anything but his eyes, the goblin just watched and waited, breathing in deeply to get all the scents around him. With a frown on his face, he took a slow step towards where they were hiding in the rocks.

"Don't make a move or a sound". The words came into her head.

Green was astonished that someone was talking to her, in her head!

"What a weird feeling", she thought.

"Not weird, it's telepathy", came Meteors' thoughts into her head. *"We have company arriving; one of the warrior dragons is nearby and enhancing our mind waves so we can all communicate".*

"Er, hello", thought Green shyly, as she had never experienced anything so fantastic.

"Well, aren't you a polite little thing" came the voice in her head, *"it's alright, I don't bite, well not other dragons anyway! Hee Hee!. Wait there, and I'll get rid of this lot for you."*

Back at the gushyberry tree, the goblins were almost drunk on the berry juice, so when one of them saw an incredible form appear in front of him on the grass; he just gaped at it.

"What are you?" he asked, getting the attention of the other two.

"It's a dragon", answered one.

"Bit big, isn't it!" said the third goblin, who was even more stupid than the others, which was quite a thing.

"Maybe, but it's only one, and they fall quicker if they are big, so I've heard."

Rising to its full height, the magnificent red dragon just stood there waiting.

"Oy Blodgy, quick, come here and see this", shouted the first goblin. "We've got ourselves a dragon, a real pretty red one."

The goblin in the clearing took a last look round and hurried off to see what was going on with his companions, giving Green and Meteor the chance to move positions.

"Just stay where you are at the moment, young 'uns, while I get rid of these nasty little blighters for you," the thought came to them both quite clearly.

So they stayed in the shelter of the rocks as ordered, wondering what was going on out by the gushyberry tree.

As the fourth goblin joined his friends, he started talking, "Oh Lawdy me, look what we have here. A poor lonesome dragon, shall we make it welcome, lads? I've never had a dragon for tea before. Heh Heh. Get it, lads. Dragon for tea, ain't I the witty one!"

Slowly they moved to surround the magnificent creature, who just stood there examining its claws.

"I will have you know you horrible little beasts. "IT" is a lady, and I have no intention of being any meal of yours", said the dragon as she continued to inspect a claw.

"Spread out, lads, and we can get it," said Blodgy, "attack when I say so, I'm sure her ladyship is too well-bred to fight. Aren't yer?"

"Oh, I promise you I won't raise a claw to you, well while you are alive, that is", replied the red dragon.

"Get her, lads."

They advanced on the dragon as she merely stood there waiting. As they got within a foot or so of her, she just shimmered and became a ball of golden-red fire. In seconds the goblins were crisply cooked and no threat to anyone.

"You can come out now, young 'uns. It is pretty safe now. Not pretty but safe", announced the dragon. Green and Meteor emerged from the wood into the clearing in front of the gushyberry tree to see the fantastic red dragon.

"Hello. Are you two alright? I am one of the warriors. Blaze is the name. I think you can guess how I got that name," she said, casually waving to the four crispy kebab goblins.

"I've come to escort you to Rainbow in Sea Valley. But first, does anyone want toasted goblin for tea? They are better than nothing, or would you prefer berries? Eat up, stretch your wings and then we will set off when you are ready."

Green looked with amazement at Blaze. "Did I just see you become a ball of fire?. It was awesome."

Preening a little, Blaze looked kindly at Green. "You're a little stunted but very talented, I reckon. Get a growth spurt on you will be fine and dandy."

Green was surprised and pleased that such an estimable dragon thought she had shown promise, and she had become telepathic as well. Sitting around whilst eating another gushyberry, Green couldn't face a crispy goblin.

"*I am not hungry enough,*" she thought. Then another thought came to her, but Blaze chuckled and answered her question before she could say anything.

"Yes, I was invisible till I let them see me, not very sporting otherwise. I would appreciate it if you didn't tell any of the other dragons about it; it's a secret weapon like the ball of fire. They all expect dragon breathing fire, and I fool them. Tell me, youngling, how did you manage to get away from the ogre? I am not reading you without your permission at the moment," Blaze said

So, Green explained being a messenger and how she had eluded the grawk.

Blaze leant forward, "what was the message you had to deliver and to whom?

Surprised, as she hadn't thought about it, the message was to Weld in the Dark Side Valley, and remembering Green reached into her scaled pocket and pulled out a sealed letter. "I don't think I will be delivering this now. Do you? As she handed it over."

Meteor had been watching and listening to them and was eager to know what the message said, but Blaze just looked at him. It was obvious they were talking mentally.

"How can you talk? Sometimes I can hear you, and I can't at other times?" Green asked them

Meteor will teach you how to block so we can't read your thoughts, but we can contact you in emergencies. When we need to be quiet, we can open up to each other and talk with our minds. It scares the lives out of the enemies when we all turn one way or fly in formation and attack without a sound. It has been described as spooky!" explained Blaze. "Now, let's see what this says. Can either of you read Ogre?"

"No," both Green and Meteor replied.

"Hmm, something you will have to learn. It is important if you get hold of messages, you can judge how dangerous a situation is when you know what the enemy is thinking, in this case, the ogres."

Slitting the pouch with a claw, Blaze started to read the message. Then she went rigid!

"Oh dragon poop!" said Meteor, "she is calling all the warriors to Sea Valley urgently, and Rainbow is seething. That's all I can tell, and they have closed me out."

All they could do was wait until Blaze sighed and relaxed.

"How are you at night flying?" she asked.

" I have done it a few times when the moon has been up," said Green.

"Good," said Blaze. "Get a drink and a couple more gushyberries down your necks, and we will be off. There's no time to waste. We've found the link to the missing younglings, and I'm afraid it is about to become nasty with the ogres!"

It took less time than fifty heartbeats till they were ready.

"OK, we're off," said Blaze. "Keep your eyes peeled and your minds linked—one on either side of me and no-nonsense. Green, if you start to tire, we will stop and rest for a short while, but we need to reach the Wooded Valley before dawn. Some of the other warriors are meeting us there. I'm sorry your welcome back to the dragons is a bit abrupt, but there is a war coming, and we haven't got time."

Through the moonlit night, they flew without stopping. Green was glad she had been a courier in all weathers, it had made her quite strong, and she kept up, though she did suspect that Blaze and Meteor were flying slower than they usually might for her benefit.

They saw the odd dragon in the distance, flying much faster.

"Messengers to other valleys, to warn them to get ready for war," said Meteor.

And so, they flew on towards daybreak and an uncertain future. . . . .

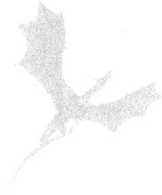

CHAPTER
3

Dan had broken over an incredible sight for Green. The place they were in was magical. There were lots of shady trees, grass meadows and then a huge area of dirt that was yellow. Sand, Meteor called it, and an enormous pond Green had ever seen was beyond that. It went on forever, as far as the eye could see, and believe me, dragons' eyes are very, very good at seeing. They had come to a halt in a small wooded area in a meadow next to the sand.

"Rest here." said Blaze, "I am just going to check in with the others, so get some sleep while you can. I will tug your brain when I want you."

"Can I go and wash in the pond?" asked Green, not quite sure what she could and couldn't do.

Blaze thought for a minute, "That pond is called the sea, and it is very salty. You obviously haven't seen it before, and it gets very deep. I suggest you clean up in the stream over there. You can play in the sea later, but don't go in without someone with you. There are many things in the sea that you will have to learn about, you will start tomorrow morning. I am sure Meteor will guide you around and help you find your way until then. Remember, if you don't know, get lost, or become confused, any of the other dragons will help, so ask!"

And with a shimmer of air, Blaze was gone.

Learning how to be a dragon, the next few days went very quickly for Green, and although some of the smaller dragons giggled when she didn't know what they were talking about, they were very good and explained things. So, Green was catching up quickly, and she had the advantage of being a powerful flier while the others in her group were still fluttering.

Greens' one great joy was the sea, and she loved to play in the waves, diving underwater and to splash the others. It was terrific to belong at last and have her own kind around her. The guardians were lovely as well unless you did something foolish or put the dragons' safety at risk, then you found out what an angry dragon looked like.

After about a week, Green realised she hadn't seen Meteor around for a while. So she asked two of the teacher guardians who were talking while watching the younglings playing in the surf.

"Excuse me, Guardian Emerald, do you know where Meteor is, please?"

Emerald looked around and smiled, "Ah, it is you, Green. Misty, do you know if Meteor is around or is he on patrol?"

The beautiful deep purple dragon answered without taking her eyes off the younglings in the water. "He went out yesterday on patrol Green; he is due back tonight before the full moon."

Frowning, Misty indicated the water well out to sea. "What do you make of that?"

Looking in the distance, they could see a large wave heading towards the shore.

"Green! Fly over there but keep high up; tell us what you see! Emerald, sound the alarm. I will get the younglings out of the water."

Green launched herself as fast as possible out to sea; keeping her height steady, she rapidly closed the distance, remembering, of course, that whatever it was, was heading towards her.

Misty ran into the water and chased the younglings onto the land. Trained to obey, they were all hurrying towards the beach.

She went beyond the younglings to protect them, unfurling her magnificent wings; she put them in the water and started to sing. It was a haunting song that made you shiver, and as it carried through the water, it got louder.

Emerald had, in the meantime, let out a dragon roar that meant it was trouble. The teacher defenders started moving all the younglings into the protection of the forest edge, the older ones helping the smaller ones. The rest of the guardians split up, half staying with the younglings to keep them safe. The others flew to the shore, rallying to the call for help.

Green now had the wave in sight. It was a churning mass of water caused by creatures about five to six feet long and the same wide. She recognised them from her sea lessons. They were Wolfcrabs, with claws that could pull you apart and a wolf-like head with wicked teeth that would rip you into bits. They were very dangerous because they could go on land and water.

"Green, what can you see?". Came the thought into her head; it was Emerald's mind speaking.

"They are wolfcrabs, big ones, about a quarter of a mile long and three or four deep, I reckon. I'm heading back now, are the younglings all out o the water yet?" replied Green.

"Yes, Green, they are in the forest defences; hurry back. Misty has summoned help as well!" answered Emerald.

"Oh! Is Rainbow coming?"

"No young one, though it is dragons. You should see signs of them coming round the headland soon."

Keeping her eyes peeled, Green flew as fast as she could to stay ahead of the approaching evil wave. As she reached Emerald and landed, Misty launched herself into the sky and circled above the beach and shallow water. Emerald told Green to get behind her and get ready to deliver messages. One of the dragons brought two great baskets of the magic chillies, which produced the fiery dragons' breath. All the guardians took two claws full and put some in their chest pouches; they then spread along the beach, chewing the chillies with relish, to a dragon they were wonderfuel.

Green decided to help and took some chillies; oh, they were beautiful to a dragon, and it was like eating chocolate. Then she felt her tummy getting warm, and with a bit of a burp, she let out a little puff of smoke. She was highly excited; she ate a few more, put some in her pouch, and did what the guardians had done. Now she was ready to be a proper dragon and fight with her dragonkin!

The wave was getting closer now, and they could see the wolfcrabs' shapes in the foam. They were scary and vicious creatures, but they had never gathered in such numbers or worked in a swarm before. Something was organising them, but what? They were swarming forward, driven by an overwhelming compulsion.

Emerald was trying to communicate with them and turn them back.

"It is just like a black void, and there are no thoughts but to destroy and feed," Emerald told the dragons. *"I cannot get through to any of them. We have no choice but to destroy them, or they will go for the younglings."*

Misty came flying in, "Help is coming, but we must hold them on the beach till then. Emerald, you take the first blast at them. With your range, it will be safe."

More guardians gathered with them, and Aura , a gold dragon, came forward. "I have some magic and a few tricks that might help," she said. "Let me stay on the frontline, and Topaz here can be a big help. She has white fire and can send some to sleep with her non-fire breath."

Topaz, a lovely pale purple dragon, said, "I am a defender. Let me do what I am supposed to. Until help comes, it is up to us guardians and defenders to keep everyone safe, so let's' get on with it. What's the plan?"

"Where are the warriors?" asked Aura.

"They have gone to Volcano Valley. There have been reports of goblins in groups, scouting around and looking for something or someone," said Green, "and I think it is me they are looking for. I feel terrible about it. Perhaps, when we've dealt with these wolfcrabs, I should go."

"Nonsense. They are always snooping around, and it's nothing to do with you; besides, we need you. You have talents that can only help us. '' said Aura. "You just don't know yet what they are, so get that silly idea out of your head now!"

She continued, "It's time to set up the battle line. I think they are nearly ashore. Ah, Misty is back, good!"

"I've been checking if that's the only attack coming at us; it's enough, though! There are about a thousand of them. I will cause the beach to rise into a huge hill barrier," said Misty, "like a castle wall that will cause a few casualties and slow them down. I suggest, Emerald, you keep your eye on the crest and use your super fire to keep it clear as long as possible. Green, can you keep everyone supplied with fire chillies? Aura, can you use some of your magic and create a deep trench on this side of the earth wall and fill it with something horrible for them? While I get some energy back, Emerald, can you ask the birds and insects to harass the wolfcrabs, buzz round their heads to distract them a bit, but not get caught? Some might fall with a bit of luck, and the others will eat them.

"Topaz, I need you to be standing by to try and send some o them to sleep as they rest the hill." went on Misty, "can your range do that? We can give it a try anyway. Everyone stays behind Emerald and Topaz; I don't want you sleeping!

"OK, dragons, we must protect the younglings and give the other dragons time to get them to safety. We have our fire and claws as our last line of defence. We all know what to do. If the fight goes against us, Green, get out of here and help the guardians with the younglings. You can fly and scout around for danger. Guardians, stay safe and protect the future till the warriors get back. Our dragon heartbeats as one, till we all meet up again, stay safe and be brave," finished Misty.

And so, the guardian dragons went into the woodland where the younglings were waiting quietly for instructions, rounded them up and set out to go to another valley for safety.

Misty, Aura, Emerald and Topaz headed towards the beach, there were other dragons as well, but their story is for another time.

They began the preparations. Misty flew up and started raising the beach into a high barrier. Aura was creating the trench, giving Misty extra ground for the wall. Green decided to place supplies of fire chillies along the defensive line for accessible collection; it would save time. All the dragons were happily munching on fire chillies and filling their pouches ready for battle. Green flew higher to get an overview and wished she hadn't. The wolfcrabs were in the surf line and starting to wade ashore.

"They are here," Green thought to the others and gave a picture of the mind so they too could see what was coming. Now they knew what they had to face.

There were a few puffs of smoke as the dragons ignited their fire, and then it was silent except for the distant surf and the click-clack of the wolfcrabs leg and the faint buzzing of insects.

Green was watching along the rim of the barrier when something caught her eye. Flying above the treeline was a grawk! Knowing the others were too busy to do anything. Green thought to Aura and told her about the grawk and would deal with it. Shooting even higher in the sky and coming out of the sun was Green's' best bet as Green had eaten some fire chillies too (she wanted to know if they were tasty) and had been practising her fire start. Praying that it would work, diving out of the sun and coming up behind the grawk with a puff of smoke, she ignited her fire.

The grawk must have sensed something because it turned and saw Green. With a vicious cry, it turned to attack, talons ready to tear and kill. Green was afraid that all these years of being a prisoner and the grawks that guarded her came into her head.

Then something snapped. Just as the grawk came close, Green let out a bellow of anger and fire for all she had suffered! Needless to say, it was one very cooked grawk that crashed into the woody growth below.

Green paused only long enough to know it was done for, or "well done for", she thought and giggled. Green flew back onto the beach to see the wolfcrabs climbing the ridge. Letting the others know she was back and OK, Green checked all the fire chilli supplies were still OK and waited with the others, quietly chewing on some more fire chillies.

As the ridge crest became crowded with wolfcrabs, everyone breathed deeply, ready for action. This was it! It was real!. Seeing the evil beasts was also terrifying as the summit became crowded. Emerald and Topaz stepped forward. The wolfcrabs were going into a frenzy, claws nipping everywhere.

Those unlucky enough to get caught by them were soon torn apart amid squeals of anger and pain being eaten alive. It was a nightmare scene with claws tearing and pulling, massive jaws crunching down. Green shuddered but dared not stop watching. As the feeding frenzy started, it was driven further by swarms of insects buzzing around their heads and blocking their vision. Still, the marauding bests surged forward, jaws and claws clacking. Then, Emerald let go with her blast of fire.

A vast swathe of fire ran along the crest, wiping out the first wolfcrabs over the ridge, and they slowly fell into the vast trench, where Topaz seared them again with white heat.

Surging off the top, more wolfcrabs moved forward, most blinded by swarms of insects; again, many fell into the trench where they fought and ate each other, tearing open shells with their wicked claws, slowing down the advance. Green was flying up and down behind the lines, ensuring the fire chillies went to those who required refills. These dragons had been scorching the wolfcrabs trying to get out of the trench.

"Can you have a look at the overall picture, please, Green?" Misty asked.

Soaring above the battle, Green realised that the wolfcrabs were even more numerous than thought. Giving Misty a mental sighting, she went even higher to provide the overall battle scene to Misty and the others.

"It's going to be dangerous if large numbers breach the barrier, with those still in the surf wanting ashore. I wonder if we can start them fighting each other, that would slow them down. Any ideas?, Green thought, and then it came to her! *"I know how; leave it to me!"*

Diving off into the woods, she went to where the baked grawk was lying, seizing it in her claws. She took off as fast as she could. Hewing on fire chillies as well, she headed for the shoreline.

"Green, be careful!" Aura silently told her.

Green made a couple of passes flying low over the swarming wolfcrabs, scorching a few with fire, but most were underwater. Aiming, Green headed towards the most significant cluster of crabs and dropped the dead (cooked) grawk into the middle of them. The sea immediately became a maelstrom of claws and jaws, tearing at the grawk and each other. Claws were ripping legs off, and jaws were pulling into the wolfcrabs next to them to get at the cooked meat. The churning water turned pink with gore and limbs; it was awful to see such cannibalism. Flying up out of reach Green spotted more churning out to sea.

"Misty, there are even more coming in from the sea about a mile out".

"We will never stop them!" Misty sighed. *"In that case, we die trying. We have to give the guardians time to get the younglings who can't fly away. And you, Green, well done! Remember, you must leave if it looks as though we are beaten. That is an order! The warriors are returning, and we just have to hold these back long enough."*

Green returned to the dragons and carried on supplying fire chillies to them. It seemed awful. Just as she had found her kin, she was to lose them. The next hour passed like a nightmare, wave after wave of wolfcrabs came ashore, only slowing to eat their fallen. The defences were covered with smoking carapaces and claws; the noise and smoke were horrendous.

Green went high again to see for all the dragons. Feeling tired and scared for all the dragons on the ground, she looked out to sea. Coming like a swathe of rainbows was a sight so welcome that Green squealed with delight.

"Look". And she passed a mental picture to the dragons, who were themselves tired, and some had been slightly injured when getting too close to the snapping claws.

Approaching at a fantastic speed came hundreds of dragons of all colours. Sparkling in the seawater, they were led by a magnificently enormous black and gold dragon. Surging into the shallow waters, they attacked the wolfcrabs from behind.

Misty called out, "Dragons go forwards; we'll catch them between us but mind you direct your fire on needle steam, so we don't hurt any of our own."

"Topaz, now is the time for you to slow them down with your sleep breath. Aura, you take command on this side of the barrier. I am going to fly to Sabre, he is the sea dragon leader, the big black and gold chap, he is my dad!" said Misty. And with that bombshell, she took off and flew over the barrier.

"OK, dragons, let's mop this lot up", said Aura. "Needlepoint fire, and we all advance in a line. Green fly around and make sure none had sneaked into this area and the edge of the woods, which was possible when all the smoke was around. Is anyone hurt? If you are, stay back and protect our backs till we can see to you. Stay alert!"

Moving forwards, the dragons formed an invincible barrier, blazing everything in their path. They slowly approached the trench.

Looking down, Aura gave the order, "Full flame! Destroy them all!"

So they did. The trench was full of baked wolfcrabs when they had finished.

"I think we can remove this now", and calling upon her magical powers; she closed the trench.

On the other side of the barrier, the sea dragons destroyed the wolfcrabs by the hundred. They too could produce fire, but of a different sort, they used a special hot chilli seaweed for theirs'. The fire was red from the dragons and very hot, and as the blast hit the wolfcrabs, they turned bright red. They were cooked in the shell, so to speak.

Misty joined her father in the onslaught on the beach.

"We need a clear shot at them now." said Sabre, "can you remove that barrier?"

Misty made the hill barrier subside, causing more chaos amongst the wolfcrabs. Trapped between two waves of dragons, the wolfcrabs had no chance. Walls of flame in two directions caught them (if you pardon the pun) in a pincer movement.

The air was thick with smoke and the redolent smell of seafood, until in a final flurry of snapping dragon jaws at all went still and quiet. The silence was astounding, with just the waves breaking on the sand.

Slowly the sea dragons advanced to the land dragons, and with a mighty roar Sabre and the others greeted their kin. Believe me, a dragon reunion is pretty chaotic, flapping wings, waving tails and delighted neck rubs. Then as everyone was sure they had greeted each other, all but Green, that is, who had held back not knowing what was happening, turned to Sabre and waited.

"It has been far too long since we gathered together", said Sabre, "we must stay awhile and get to know each other better. My brother and the warriors are nearly here, so let's set up a feast ready. We have plenty to go around. It's baked crab for dinner! We can get some gushyberries; it's a long time since I've had some, and any other treats we can find, rabbits perhaps; I am partial to a rabbit or grawk."

"Which reminds me." continued Sabre, "who was the brave soul who brought the baked grawk to distract the wolfcrabs?"

Aura turned and nudged Green forward, "This is Green. She hasn't got her adult name yet, and she escaped from the ogres and has been a blessing to us all!"

"That's right," said Topaz, "she even taught herself to fly."

Green shrunk as small as she could with embarrassment.

"Didn't do anything the others haven't done," she said, wishing she could curl up. All the dragons were looking at her curiously.

Topaz put a wing reassuringly over Green's shoulder. "Come and meet Sabre. He doesn't bite, you know, well not dragons anyway."

Sabre bowed his great head and gave Green a tremendous toothy smile. "I bet you know where all the best gushyberry trees are. Shall you and I find some? And leave this lot to clear up!"

There was a sound of heavy wing beats, and onto the beach area came the warriors led by Rainbow.

"Thank goodness everyone is ok, Rainbow said. "Misty told me you had arrived, Sabre. Thank you. We got here as fast as we could"

Then Sabre and Rainbow flew at each other and proceeded to wrestle and roll around, as brothers do! Delighted to see each other, the dragons' grins were as big as crocodiles.

Still unsure, Green started to go to the back of the large group of dragons when a voice in her head said, *I thought we were going for gushyberries? Just give me a minute, then we will be off.*

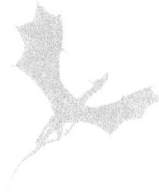

CHAPTER

4

So, amidst much good humour and jostling they flew off in search of the gushyberrys and any other "Treats" they could find. Green had the forethought to take a large net with her to make carrying easier, but didn't know how much it would be needed!

While they were out Sabre touched Green's mind and they 'talked' of many things. He knew about her time with the ogres, Rainbow had told him about her story, but there were a few gaps he wanted to know about. Like the layout of Welds' castle, when she had been there and what it was made of. Lots of seemingly silly questions.

"Look! What's that?" said Green indicating a mound of blue on the ground.

Flying down towards it Sabre said "Stay above me, flying around and keep your eyes open! It could be a trap, I will look."

As Sabre approached the shape it moved slowly. It was an injured blue dragon, its wings were staked through into the ground and its tail tied to a big rock.

"Help me please before they come back," said the dragon, "my name is Skye."

"Green, is it all clear up there?" asked Sabre. "If so, come and help, but keep your eyes open and your smell well tuned in."

Gliding in, Green landed, wincing at the sight of the damaged winds.

Sabre said, "While I hold him still use your teeth to pull the stakes out." Then to Skye, "Who did this? And how did you get caught?"

Green's nose twitched as she hurried to undo Skye's tail. "Goblins," she said. "Lots of them by the smell they have left. Can you fly?"

"No," replied Skye, "my wings are numb."

"Quickly," said Sabre, "the next Skye, climb onto it, I will fly us out of here. Green do you have any fire chillies left? If so, chew them quickly and act as rearguard while I carry the net"

As his legs were also numb, Skye rolled onto the net. Sabre gathered up the corners, and slowly and gently rose into the air. Green did the same, circling round to protect them, and then off they went.

"Phew, that was close" she thought, "Look down there!"

Swarming below them were hundreds of goblins, running around looking for Skye.

Then they were spotted and a flurry of arrows were fired into the air, naturally they fell short, and even Sabre chuckled at the sight of the goblins trying to dodge their own falling arrows.

"Let's get out of here and warn the others," said Sabre, "I have told Rainbow and he is assembling the warriors, but they don't know if there are any more groups like this. We have to keep the younglings safe from any other raiding parties."

It took a steady time to fly back, so that Skye did not suffer more than necessary. On reaching the Sea Valley they slowly lowered the net to where many willing dragons were waiting to help.

"Goblins, hoards of the little blighters," said Sabre. "This is Skye, thanks to Greens's sharp eyes we were able to get him away."

"Right," said Rainbow, "everyone is to eat their fill, we don't know when we will have time again, and it is a shame to waste this baked wolfcrab. Looks like we have another battle to come. Does it not seem strange to you Sabre, all these attacks are coming at the same time!"

"You said you had intercepted a message, was it anything to do with this? How did you get it? asked Sabre.

"Green, she was being used as a carrier by the ogres, until we rescued her. She still had an undelivered message, perhaps that is the reason for all this," mused Rainbow.

Noticing all the interested dragons had gathered round listening, they moved away from the crown and continued the discussion.

"I think Green was the catalyst. She is more important to this than we know" Rainbow finished.

"You know you cannot keep calling her Green, she has more than earned her adult name," said Sabre. "Has she been to the Crystal Valley yet?"

"No," said Rainbow, "we were to go onto there when we left the Sea Valley. She had never seen anything like the valleys, so we were trying to give her some pleasure to widen her horizons. One thing we must do while we are together is 'The Mind Link' with Blaze here and the other telepaths, plus your people, we must make everyone, young and old telepathic,so we can be alerted if there is anything wrong."

!I agree, and no time like the present." said Sabre. "What about Skye, do we include him; we don't know where he is from yet?"

"So let's ask him," sid Rainbow reading the way back to where Skye was being tended to. "I think we will question after the 'Link' that way we will know the truth."

Green was putting freezeweed on Skye's wounds. "It will stop the pain and speed up the healing for you." she told Skye.

"Thank you," replied Skye, "it feels better already. It works fast."

"Right dragons," called Rainbow. "Sabre, please go to the other side with the sea telepaths."

When everyone had gathered between the two lines of telepathic dragons, Rainbow told them what was going to happen.

"You will all feel a queer sensation, a bit like pins and needles for a couple of seconds, it's just like a bee buzzing." he told the younglings who had returned, "then you will hear us speak in your heads. When you hear us clearly raise your wings to the sky."

With their wings out to the sides, the telepathic dragons touched each other and started a strange humming noise, the same with the dragons on the other side, until a resonant harmony filled the air, and slowly one after another the dragons in the centre started raising their wings. It was a spectacular sight, every colour and shade of the rainbow, glittering and shining in the sunlight. Even Skye was affected and he managed to lift his halfway up.

"Dragons Roar" thought Rainbow, and a myriad of voices road skyward! *"Dragons Silent"* thought Sabre and a quiet fell over Sea Valley.

Rainbow said "All of you experienced telepaths take groups and teach them how to use this power now. Sabre, Green and I have to go to the Crystal Valley, so be aware and look after each other. Blaze, I am leaving you in charge, look at your defences. Get patrols out and I want everyone to know where each other is, No straying off younglings, this is where you start to be dragons for real. Green, will you come to your adult ceremony in the Crystal Valley?"

Green nodded, too full of emotions to speak. Finally she was going to Crystal Valley and find out who she really is.

CHAPTER
5

S o, into the evening flew Rainbow, Sabre and green, heading towards the setting sun.

Over different valleys they went until Rainbow though to Green, *"Bear left till we reach those trees on the other side of the valley, we will rest there tonight."*

Slowly they descended on to a meadow in front of the trees, with a stream meandering through it.

"Do you think there will be any rabbits," thought Sabre, *"I'm feeling a bit peckish!"*

"It should be safe enough here," said Rainbow, "have a scout around first though, keep quiet and keep your wits about you!"

"Green there is a gushyberry tree over there, get yourself some to eat and then try and get some sleep if you can."

But, Green wasn't too tired and she had a lot of questions in her head. Turning towards Rainbow she realised that he must have heard her jumbled thoughts as he was looking at her with a smile and a raised brow.

"You want to know what the Crystal Cavern is, and what will happen?" he said. "Settle down and I will do what I can to explain."

"The cavern is huge, big enough for fifty dragons, and in it are the golf and jewels which our ancestors have collected through the centuries. They are beautiful and shiny and glitter like sunlight on water, but the walls and roof are covered in crystals that reflect the colour of the jewels and the light like a giant moving rainbow, flickering back and forth!"

"You mean it is like you dancing", chuckled Green.

"That would be a funny sight indeed," said Sabre as he joined them, "but it is beautiful beyond description, and it has special powers as well!"

"When you go in there, you will stay for one night alone," continued Rainbow, "don't worry we will be guarding the entrance, and that is the only way in. You will be quite safe."

"But what happens?" asked Green.

"Ah! Now , it's different for each of us." explained Rainbow, "some just go to sleep and wake up next morning knowing their adult name and knowing what they are going to do with their lives."

"Others are given skills, and some have visions of the future, but when you come out you will be an adult dragon and be marked as such in some way."

"Rainbow here was destined to be the leader of all the dragon clans," said Sabre. "Our King I suppose some wou;ld call him, and he carries the colour of every dragon and clan, you won't know this but he can just be one colour as well,as and when circumstances need it!"

"Enough about me, this is Greens' time," said Rainbow. "Come daybreak we will enter the cave and teach you what each of the gems are, and what magic they enhance."

"May I ask." said Green, looking from one to the other, "Why are you black then Sabre?"

Laughing Sabre explained, "I am a Sea Dragon and although I can live on land, and you could live in the sea, the light underwater, especially where it is deep and dark, is very different, I am actually multi-coloured like Rainbow, but it doesn't show in sunlight, just as

Rainbow is black underwater. You will understand better tomorrow. The cavern will teach you everything you need to know!"

"Do all dragons come here?" Green queried.

"Yes, it's a sort of 'Rite of Passage', some come earlier than others," said sabre. "We were headed this way, unfortunately when we got your call for help. Sea dragons all come together here and meet up at some time, it's like a really big party. Since we live in the seven seas we don't meet up very often. Time for a rest young dragon, you have a big day in front of you, and I for one am not getting any younger! So take pity on an old dragon and sleep!"

Laughing, Green did as Sabre asked, and soon fell asleep.

Sitting quietly for a while, lost in their own thoughts, just enjoying each other's company before the world and reality intruded, they watched the stars. The two brothers slowly relaxed.

"OK", said Sabre, "what did you really want a conclave of dragons for? The rest by the way are following on at the younglings pace, I just came ahead with my warriors."

After due thought to organise his words Rainbow began; "Young Green was a courier for the ogres, she was hatched from a stolen egg and kept prisoner. She had a message to deliver when we got to her, and there have been goblins and grawks searching for her ever since. The message was to Weld, and had an ancient spell or recipe in it which was 'How to take the Dragons' powers as your own!' That was bad enough but the main ingredient was a young dragon, to be eaten by Weld for the power. Green was meant to be a test to see if the spell worked, But, the major factor was the reference to, 'The other hatched eggs and the white dragon protecting them' that Weld has."

Sabre jumped up, and in his agitation unfurled his wings and spikes. "How can you sit there so calm when we know where \pearl and the eggs are?"

Rainbow answered quietly. They are younglings now, the same as Green. We know they are alive and that Pearl is with them, but where, that is the question. We've searched high and low on Decagon for them, the only place left is the Dark Side. I couldn't take the chance of him thinking we know, and killing them all. But if he wants power through his spell, their time is running short!"

"That's why Green is here isn't it, to find out what her destiny is." Sabre said quietly.

"True, I'm very fond of her, she is brave and resourceful and a minx. But I believe she is the key to rescuing Pearl and the younglings."

"It must have broken your heart the night she and the eggs were taken," said Sabre.

"I've wondered how they did it without her raising the alarm," continued Rainbow. "We lost two good warriors that night. I know it was goblin poison that killed them, but why take Pearl?"

"The eggs were near their hatching time, I can only suppose that she was taken to look after them, and the only thing that could have stopped her giving the alarm would be the threat of breaking the eggs and killing the young ones. Pearl would want to keep them alive, and trust me to find them. It's taken too long; I've failed her Sabre."

"Rubbish! We know they are alive and where they probably are. You've only failed if we don't get them out in time."

And each went back to their thoughts.

Slowly, the hint of light crept over the horizon, and as the sun slowly came up, Rainbow turned to Sabre, "Are you in with us brother mine, it could be a costly fight!"

Sabre looked at the rising sun and nodded.

"If we don't stop Weld, he will kill as many dragons as possible for their power, and then the rest will be at risk. We must put an end to this forever and get our younglings and Pearl back. Perhaps we should enter the cave too. It has given answers before when needed. Now about them rabbits?"

When Green woke up, it was to see rainbow and Sabre with half a dozen cooked rabbits.

"Have you two been asleep?" she asked.

"There's some rabbit left for you, you must be hungry. I cooked it so we could use it later if needed, said Sabre.

"Thank you," said Green, helping herself to a big fat one, "I'm starving, this is delicious," she mumbled with her mouth full.

"Time to go," said Rainbow, "don't be worried, it's a wonderful experience, and Sabre and I will be outside. We will be coming in to join you a bit later, but the first bit is for you alone."

After a careful look to make sure no one or anything was around, they flew with Rainbow to a side of the valley that was all rocky terrain. Deep into a fissure they went. In single file, to the entrance of a cavern. It was large, big enough for them to fly into and then it opened out into another cave. Landing, Green was very nervous.

"Are you sure you won't come in with me? You said you were coming in later anyway," Green said in a shaky voice.

Rainbow put his wing over Green. "It's alright, but you need to see the beauty and magic on your own. It is truly awe inspiring. But if you are afraid, shout, and we will come to you."

Green set off slowly into the huge cavern and gradually vanished from sight.

"Wait for it," said Sabre, "anytime now!"

Sure enough, after a minute or two, all you could hear was "Ooohh, Oh and other exclamations of awe.

"Oh my goodness!" came echoing out as a whisper. Looking at each other and chuckling, the two brothers sat down to wait.

Inside the cavern, Green had found all sorts of treasures piled high. But it was the crystal walls and roof that astounded her. "My goodness!" she said again, there were glorious colours everywhere. Green had been told to go into the centre of the cavern where a large freshwater pool sat. So following instructions she went to the pool and entered it slowly. The water was soft and almost warm. She had never been in a big pool before and revelled in being able to splash and unfurl her wings in the water, bliss! Cavorting around like a dolphin, Green swam to the opposite side where a small waterfall fed the pool. Taking a tentative sip she found it was beautifully fresh and sweet, so she drank her fill.

Stepping out of the pool she went to a large flat stone that overlooked the treasure stored there, and sat down. Slowly her eyelids began to close and she drifted into an enchanted dreamlike state.

About an hour later she awoke from the dream state and stretched. Surprised, she noticed a small pile of stones by her feet. They were the most incredible colour she had ever seen. Picking them up she placed them in her pouch.

Then she went to one wall that was almost a mirror and looked, seeing a sleek bright green shimmering dragon. Stretching her wings, she saw they were too shimmering with glorious scales, looking just like the stones. A soft whisper, like a gentle breeze, came to her.

"Your name is 'Peridot' from now on, but close friends will call you 'Perri'. This is a sign of affection, accept it for what it is."

"Peridot. I have a name, a real name, and it's mine!"

Hurrying to the entrance to tell Rainbow and Sabre, she felt a little bit awkward and then it dawned on her, She was bigger, she had grown into herself! Hearing steps in the cavern Rainbow and Sabre stood, and were astounded at the dragon now before them.

"My lady dragon, welcome, and by what name should we call you?" Rainbow inquired politely.

"My name is Peridot, my lord," said Peridot, and then burst into a fit of giggles, "but please, both of you, call me Perri."

Embracing her her with their wings the two warriors were delighted at the happy dragon before them

"We are going into the cavern. We need some answers and guidance," said Rainbow. "Will you keep watch for us please?" We are vulnerable in the cavern that's why we waited for you outside. I don't think this valley has been found, but, with grawks flying the goblins everywhere, it is just a matter of time."

Perri sat herself just inside the fissure cave so she could see, but not be seen, as Rainbow and Sabre entered the cavern. Watching the valley with interest, there were Sabres favourites, rabbits, by the hundred, romping in the grassland below, they were funny to watch. Thinking about it she realised she had never been able, before, to just sit and watch. Suddenly all of the rabbits scattered in panic. Alert now, Perri stayed in the shadows looking for the danger. Then she saw it, a shadow slowly flying over the grassland. It wasn't big enough to be a dragon, it had to be a grawk, and the shadow made it quite clear that there was a goblin on its back.

Slowly backing into the cave, but where she could still see the shadow gliding around, Perri debated what to do. Stay out of sight, call the dragons in the cave, or, go kill the grawk and the goblin.

The trouble with that was, there may be more around and that would give them away. Deciding just to watch and wait was hard, but it was the wisest course, until Sabre and Rainbow came back out.

CHAPTER
6

Meanwhile. . .

Back in Sea Valley, Skye was overwhelmed with the kindness he was being shown, though he was fully aware that someone was with him or watching him all the time. He was just so glad that Topaz had stitched his wings up where he had been staked, and that freezing cream was wonderful at taking the pain away. He knew it was only while he recovered, then they would ask questions.

Topaz and Blaze were watching some younglings frolic in a large pool.

"So what are your readings on Skye?" asked Blaze. "Any idea where he's from? I thought we were the last dragons."

"He wasn't telepathic till the dragon roar. '' said Topaz, "now he is much easier in his own mind that we won't hurt him. I haven't probed. I think you need to ask the questions Blaze!"

"No time like the present I sup[pose. Hopefully we will have some answers by the time the others get back." replied Blaze.

Blaze then sent a mental message to Meteor asking him to bring Skye to the pool area.

"WE must have patrols out goblin hunting," said Blaze. "I'm going to ask Misty if she and the sea dragons can take care of that. Imagine sabre being her dad, I always knew she was part sea dragon."

"Does Sabre have a mate/" asked Topaz.

"Yes, her name is Coral. Misty's mother was killed in one of the ogre battles. He waited till Misty grew up and joined us land dragons, then he found Coral. She was injured and he rescued her from some savage 'mer' man, but that's a long story. They have not talked about it much but they bonded. Coral is with the other sea dragons following behind Sabre and his warriors. They can only go as fast as the younglings and will be here in a few days."

"I've sent Emerald to meet them and take them to Rainbow Valley. It will give them time to rest up, and us time to plan, there are now developments."

Meteor ambled into where Skye was. "Blaze would like to talk to you by the large pond. I'll take you there. I am Meteor by the way. It's going to be fun to have another male to lark with. We can go fishing when you are fitter. All the other lads are on Volcano duty at the moment. I've done my stint on that. At the moment I am Rainbows   aide, I'm a warrior." he said proudly, leading Skye by the path to the pool.

"Hello Skye," said Blaze. "We need to find out what's happening here, so could you answer a few questions please?"

Sitting down, Skye told them his story.

"I am from a land across the ocean, I was our strongest flier, so I got the job. It's about five flying days from here in the West, there are about eight hundred of us, all ages and we need to escape from where we are. I was sent to see if we were the last dragons, and if there was anywhere we could move to and settle. \\\You are the first dragons I've seen apart from our clan. I can't tell you how happy I am to find you, and that you ate kind as well. Can you help us please?"

Blaze looked surprised. "Of course we will help. We are dragon kin; we all help each other. But, what are you escaping from?Is it possible it will follow you here? Do we need to be battle ready?"

"Right," said Skye, "the danger is drought. There were streams and lakes, rivers as wide as the eye could see. But in the last few years they have started to dry up and slowly our land is becoming a desert. We don't know why, the only thing left for us is to find a new home. Can you help us please? Another problem is we have more males than females and that is causing tension as well."

"You could have some of ours." piped up Meteor, "we have lots more females than males."

"That's enough!" Blaze said. ")Of course we will help. Rainbow and Sabre will be back soon and we can work out what to do. Are any of your dragons telepathic?"

"Only the older ones" said Skye, "they wouldn't teach us how to do it, so they could stay in charge."

"Ah." said Blaze "like that is it. Well, we can soon sort that out. If we contact them, will they be cooperative or want to take over if we bring them here? What's your opinion Skye. You know these dragons."

Startled at being asked his opinion, Skye thought for a while. "I think they would be all friendly and cooperative, but they wouldn't want to lose power, so would be looking for ways to take over. They are not like you, asking each other's opinions and sharing ideas. I like your way better than just being ordered around."

"Well," said Topaz, "it's very difficult to be rotten and to plot when you are telepaths. Even if you close your mind we can still tell if someone is mad or being spiteful. The first thing after making contact is to use the dragon roar to make everyone telepathic, then they can start integrating with us and the elders can't start plotting. What say you Blaze?"

"Good scheme! And if they don't know we are all telepaths still it is too late even better! Arf arf!! I love a battle of wits. We would just have to make sure that there was no contact with Weld a co. One thing," continued Blaze, "there will be a dragon gathering tonight when Rainbow gets back. You will be needed, so Meteor will stay with you. L know he is dying to go fishing, have you ever done that? No! Why not go and see what you can catch/"

So, the two young male dragons went off quite happily to go fishing. This involved going into the water and chasing the fish for dinner.Great fun if you are a dragon, (that is assuming Skye could swim, he will soon learn if Meteor is

around).

"Right," said Blaze, "we need a valley as far away from the dark side as possible, which do you recommend?"

"Here in Sea Valley,! Said Topaz without hesitation, "it's got everything that will be wanted. Water, food, forests and caves for shelter, and only one way in and out which can be guarded till we know if they will have troublemakers. But I think I will ask Emerald to get the dolphins and whales to make sure they stay there; we don't want them to realise we are sea dragons as well."

"We can all move across to Secret Valley. It will put us between the newcomers and Ice Valley and be handy for food from the Herd and Pasture Valley for both sides, then we and the sea dragons in Rainbow Valley and Secret Valley will be on hand if they are a problem, finished Topaz.

"Perfect, let's get every one sorted; as the guardians to see to that please, I was thinking, for the younglings we could pop them into nets like we did Skye, that way they can all be transported together by air and we can have them all over there before dark," said Blaze.

"What a good idea," said Topaz, "I don't know why it hasn't been done before? The younglings will think it's a great adventure."

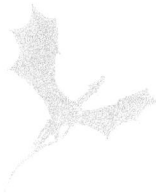

CHAPTER
7

Back in Crystal Valley, Peri was still on guard in the cave. She kept looking back into the cavern to warn the other two about the goblins. At last she heard footsteps coming from behind her. "Thank goodness you are back; there are grawks and goblins out there. I've counted three sets so far; they are searching the valley."

Carefully looking out Rainbow watched for the grawks, after a while he asked, "Did you see goblins on all the grawks?"

"Yes," replied Peri.

"In that case the goblins are on foot looking around," continued Rainbow. "We need to be careful they don't find the cave, move a bit further back into the deeper shadows. We cannot leave while they are around. Sabre, you know they must not leave this valley alive!"

"So, we must sneak up on them, perhaps in the dark?" said Sabre. "We must take the grawks out as well, and leave no trace."

"Pity we are low on fire," said Rainbow, "we could have scorched them and dumped them in Volcano Valley. Oh dear, caught in an eruption blast."

Peri listened and watched the entrance. "I was supplying the fire chillies during the big fight," she said. "I had just loaded my pouch up when it finished, I've got loads here," and tipping them onto a flat rock, she asked "is this enough for us three?" You know it sounds silly but I think they are looking for me," Peri continued, "that letter must be more important than we thought, but they won't recognise me, unless they are just looking out for a green dragon, is that possible?"

"It is indeed, they aren't very bright, '' said Rainbow, "and it does seem a bit strange then straying so far from the dark side. I think you are right Peri, How can we use this."

"Well," said Peri, "how about we load up on fire and as it gets towards dusk, I go and sit on that rock just outside the cave. Then you and Sabre can come and scorch them, or, wait till they camp for the night. They always light a fire, I think they are scared of the dark and I could land and distract them there. Then you can come out of the dark and catch them all at once! I can tell you when I land if they are all there and they certainly won't know I am a fire dragon and can zap them!"Rainbow and Sabre were chuckling, "My we have got a proper little warrior on our hands, when did you get to be so devious and bloodthirsty!"

"When I found out they wanted to eat me! And I am not that little now, and yes, I do want to be a warrior."

Sabre looked at her and said, "I am sorry if you thought we were laughing at you, but you are magnificent for a new dragon adult, and yes, you are a warrior in my eyes,"

Peri blushed, "Oh! I'm sorry that it was a bit rude of me to shout at you both, but I got mad!"

"Nonsense, always stick up for yourself." said Rainbow.

"And think for yourself as well as others," added Sabre. "So, what are we going to do?"

Rainbow whispered, "Well first of all let's get these fire chillies eaten, and then we will have to deal with the goblin that is heading towards us!"

"What if we go into the outer cave," said Peri, "you cover me with dust and dirt and I curl up and pretend to be scared and defenceless. Then you can let them take me prisoner and I can pretend to be glad they have come to rescue me, that way we'll know where their camp is and how many there are."

"I like it", said Sabre, "and you Rainbow, what do you think?"

"I don't think we have much choice; we must keep the Crystal Cavern secret. OK, let's get you all dirtied up! Your fire level ok? Right, remember to stay in touch with us with the mental link. Blame the big storm for blowing you here, and you have been nursing a hurt wing, that's why you couldn't fly out of here. Now it is better, but you didn't know where you were or which way to fly."

So scared but excited as well, Peri went into the outer cave and Sabre and Rainbow flapped their wings and blew dust and dirt on Peri till she looked positively dull. Then she curled up and pretended to be asleep.

Sabre and Rainbow retreated into the cavern shadows, they waited patiently.

"Why that stupid bird can't fly up here I don't know," grumbled the goblin. "Down draughts indeed!. So, I've got to climb and check every bloomin' cave. Ridiculous I call it!"

Reaching the cave entrance, the goblin called out, "Cooee, anybody there?"

Imagine his shock when a feeble little voice answered, "Hello! Have you come to help me please?"

"Oh lawks! There's summat in there, now what do I do," exclaimed the surprised goblin.

"Well you could help me for a start! Have you any water please?"

"It talks! Lordy me. Well seeing as how I don't know who I am talking to, I'm not coming any nearer!"

"My name is P.... Green, I've been stuck in here with a hurt wing and I am lost and afraid, you are not going to harm me, are you? Please help me!"

Feeling in charge of the situation the goblin stepped further into the cave.

"Now don't you worry I will help you. You just come with old Farty here, I will take you back to our camp, we've been looking for you, young 'un."

"Oh, how wonderful!" gushed Peri, "it's so lovely to know someone cares about me! I have been fed up with eating berries and worms, and having no one to talk to."

"Never mind you come along now, you will be fine and dandy. Maybe if we pass a stream on the way to the camp you can have a drink and clean some of that dirt off, don't want the ogres thinking we haven't looked after you, do we? And the old Farty here doesn't want any blame!"

So, they set off from the cave into the valley. Peri kept an eye out for Rainbow and Sabre, but she never saw a trace of them. They had been travelling for about an hour when they found a stream.

"There you are missy, as I promised. Now get yourself a drink and a bath, you will feel much better. I will just be over there having forty winks, shout if you need me."

When Peri had her drink, she waded into the stream and started along it.

"Oy! Where are you going?2 asked Farty.

"Just down here the water is deeper and I can get my wings under," replied Peri.

"No further then, how can I look after you if I can't see you!" came the reply from Farty.

Slowly washing the dust off Peri thought to Rainbow, *"Are you here?"*

"I am behind you in the bushes. We split up to find the goblins' grawk.. Sabre will take it out, one less to deal with! Are you OK?"

"Fine. How am I going to explain my sparkle?" asked Peri.

"Blame it on the diamond dust, it must have polished your scales, they are daft enough to believe it." laughed Rainbow. *"When I flew over I saw their camp. It is about ten minutes flying time from here, the stream runs by it. If you have to, get into the water and head upstream to this*

glade. We will meet you. But mind link when you get there, then we can see and hear what you do."

"Oy Missy! Haven't you finished yet?" came Fartys' voice, "It's time to move on"

Peri stepped out of the water. "My Aunties whiskers! What have you done? You're all sparkly and bright, you glitter!"

"Why so I do," answered Peri, "I wonder how that's happened? Perhaps the dust polished my scales! Was it diamond dust? Do you know? Or maybe it's something in the water? It's pretty anyway!"

"Come on, it's time we got going." and setting off at a brisk pace, Farty led the way.

It took about an hour to get to the camp on foot. Peri was sure he had lost his way a couple of times, but they eventually arrived. And what a dirty scruffy camp it was. The only welcoming thing was the big fire burning in the centre. It was both light and heat and as the sun was starting to set, it was getting cold. Going closer to the fire Peri counted the goblins , there were five , and four grawks. Leaping up with a startled shout they rushed forward.

"Hello," said \peri. "Farty said you were friendly when he found me, it's good of you to search for me!"

Well, they stopped dead, not sure what to do. No one had ever thanked them for hunting them before! Then Farty strolled into the clearing.

"Ah you see, I've found Missy here in a cave." Looking at his leader he winked. "It seems she was blown here by that bad storm and hurt a wing. Can't fly and was lost as well, and here we are to rescue her. Isn't that good!"

The goblin leader who was a little bit smarter than the others asked "What is your name?"

"Green," Peri answered. "I am a messenger for the ogres who live in the valley next to \Lord Weld. It was so kind of the ogres to send out a search party to find me."

"Is she real?" whispered one of the other Goblins.

"They said she wasn't very bright," answered his partner. "Doesn't know anything but flying messages, nice and polite though and very shiny, we won't lose her easily. Ha ha!"

"Did they send all of you out to look for me?" asked Peri, "or did you all just meet up here? I've never had so many look for, or care about me." she asked fishing for numbers.

Puffing his chest out, with his own importance, the leader announced, "We was a speshul chosen group to search everywhere. We've been searching for weeks now, but we've found you and i will get promoted for it!"

"How nice for you. W said peri. "What will you do next then?"

"The team and I will go to the south and be on duty killing mermaids and mermen, 'horrible fishy people, not even nice to eat, but at least we'll be away from his lordship and his tantrums!"

"Now is the time to leave," said Sabre mentally to Peri, *"We have you covered, tell them you want to pee or something and head for the stream, you know where to meet us."*

"Excuse me sir," said Peri quietly to the leader, "I have to go pee, where do I go, over in the woods?"

"No," he answered, "we don't want you getting lost, go into the bushes by the stream over there and be quick about it!"

Moving quickly Peri headed in the direction she had been told to go, and entered the bushes moving straight through them to the stream, slipping quietly into the water, she swam upstream very easily and soon arrived at the glade that was the meeting place, and settled down to wait. She was settled down by some bushes waiting for Rainbow and sabre to contact her, when she heard a noise.

Pulling back into the shade she messaged Sabre *"Are you at the clearing?"*

"No," came back the answer, *"be prepared to fight, one got away, we are on our way."*

Watching carefully, she saw a movement by the stream. Someone was coming her way. Turning on her dragon night vision, she saw a goblin. It was the leader of the group. Was he hunting her, or was he trying to escape?

Knowing what she must do, Peri stepped forward into the light, "Are you looking for me? She asked.

Jumping in the air, the goblin turned to face her. "You. I should have known you were trouble. Well I'm going to kill you, at least the others will be avenged!", and running at her he held a large curved knife in his hand.

Peri knew the moment had come. It was kill or be killed. Taking a deep breath, she activated her fire and sent a blast wave of white-hot fire at the goblin, and he was no more. She didn't feel guilty.after all, they were going to kill her or even worse, take her back to the ogres to be eaten.

It's survival, she said to herself sternly, just don't use your power unless it is to protect.

"Well done Peri," came the voice of Rainbow in her head. *"We are not wanton killers;we just protect our own and ourselves. There is not a creature in this world that doesn't do the same."*

And, with a mighty draught from their wings Rainbow and Sabre landed, and putting their wings around her they held her close.

"Now we can rest here, or start back to the others and rest when we get back!"

"We need to rejoin them as soon as possible ," said Peri, "the visions I had in the cave tell me some great trouble is approaching. You two are needed badly. Have you been in contact with the others yet?"

"Yes," said Rainbow, "and the move to Secret Valley is completed. Patrols are up and Volcano Valley is activated, so let's just get back and ready ourselves for the next problem, which will be to rescue the younglings.

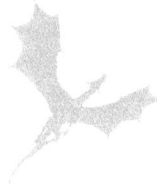

CHAPTER
8

Blaze had transferred the whole dragon kin to Secret Valley overnight, and left just a few volunteers behind to remove any traces of occupancy in Sea Valley. As dawn broke, and sunlight flooded the valley, turning it from a golden glow to a lush paradise. Everyone had eaten and settled down to rest, keeping a watchful eye on the ever-energetic younglings.

When Rainbow, Sabre and Peridot arrived back it caused quite a stir, especially Peri who was the centre of attention amongst the younger dragons. She was rather pleased at her new look; she had seen herself in the lake as they entered the valley and thought she looked quite grand. Vanity was soon forgotten though, when Rainbow called for a 'Dragon Roar', something important was up!

"As you know, my beloved dragons, Peri, that's her adult name, had a letter in her keeping when she joined us, and a bit of luck it was too! It's from the ogres to Weld, and gives the recipe for cooking dragons, in order to power a spell to take all their powers and strength. Weld wants to do this. It is he who stole our eggs, and he has Pearl prisoner!"

At this announcement, all the dragons gasped in horror at the sheer evil of this plot, and an uproar broke out wanting vengeance.

"Quiet", called Rainbow, "we must go into this with calm heads and cold hearts, our younglings, as they will be now, will be slaughtered on the spot. For some reason Pearl cannot communicate with us. I suspect iron is being used to block her power and strength. I need you adults to explain to our younglings here, that they must obey every order and not mess about if given one. Lives will depend on it!"

"The sea dragons are on this quest with us," continued Rainbow, and Coral and the others will be here soon. We have also discovered a distant dragon colony, where Skye has come from to ask for our help. Skye has also asked to become one of our family permanently. He is now your brother dragon, and will be welcomed as such by us all. I want you all to go into your groups and discuss ideas for rescuing our dragons. We will meet here as the sun starts to set. Oh! And, no matter how silly you think it is, listen to the younglings, they sometimes have very simple solutions" finished Rainbow.

Meeting up with Sabre, Blaze, Misty, Rae, Emerald, Peri, Meteor, Topaz along with Aura and Skye, they walked a short distance out of earshot. "Close your minds for a moment," said Rainbow, "I don't want this heard by any but you, the Inner Circle. I have included Skye, because I think he could help us."

"Anything", said Skye, looking eager.

"Have you been taught to block thoughts?" asked Rae.

"Yes, Meteor told me how and we practised, and he told me how to block goblin smell," replied Skye. "What else can I learn?"

"Depending on what ideas come up we have some things to find out," said Rainbow. !I've tried to list them, but please come in with your own ideas as well!"

We need to find the exact location of Welds' castle and who or what's in it. Are there any allies around there?"

Look for guards, how many and routines and timings.

Try and find ways in. The sneakier the better!

Find out where the younglings are, and are they fit to escape?

Find out if Pearl is with the younglings, or is she kept separate and if so. where?

"One thing to remember, if you come in on this team you will be warriors and nothing stops the rescue. So, if you have any doubts, say so, no-one will think any less of you. You will have another equally important job," finished Rainbow.

Aura suggested, "Nets, that's worked well for us before. We can use them to get the younglings out and away quickly, so we will need a team of guardians and defenders just for that job, present company excepted."

"We could do with eyes and ears on the inside, I can be invisible, and go and do a recce without being seen," said Blaze. "We also need the layout and exits in case we get rumbled."

"And a rendezvous base in a safe area," Sabre chipped in.

"What about escaping via the Volcano Valley," continued Blaze, "they won't expect that will they? And it is very close. You will need to have the defenders who are with the nets start practising with heavier weights, as we don't know how many will be airlifted, or if they can fly.." finished Blaze.

"My dragons can help there," said Sabre, "they can overfly the net teams and help defend them and also help with the airlift, and then, be a rearguard against attack from the air. We don't know where the goblins who fly the grawks are. In the castle? Where? It's vital we find out!"

Rainbow shook his head, "There are so many things that cannot be predicted; but lives are at stake!"

While this discussion was going on, a young dragon called Spike went to Blaze.

"May I have a word, my lady? I don't know if it means anything, and I have told no-one, but a few times I'lve been trying to avoid the younglings and teachers, sorry. They walked right past me, at first I thought I was just good at hiding, but as time went on I realised they couldn't see me. That's when I tried doing it on purpose, can you tell, if at all, can I be invisible and how to control it. It must help if there are two of us to spy out the castle and as I am only half your size I can sneak into dungeons, they always have narrow stairs."

"Hmmm, so you think you can disappear eh! Come on then, while they are all plotting, we will have a little trial run, but, whatever I teach you, you will tell no-one. So come on."

Launching into the air Blaze followed by Spike flew off for a quieter area. As they flew off, Sabre and Rainbow looked at each other and smiled. "Told you," said Sabre.

After a while the discussion slowly petered out and catching up as brothers do, they talked for a while about family and friends, then Rainbow said, "Sabre, if I don't come back and pearl is gone, you and Coral must take over as dragon Lord and Lady. I have already spoken to Blaze and the council so there will be no problem, except you will have to give up your sea life. Have you got a replacement ready, just in case?"

"Yes," said Sabre, "but it won't come to that, and on the same subject, Misty is my successor so she will have to find a helpmate eventually, perhaps these new dragons will have a few choices for her, who knows?"

Sending out a mental thought for Meteor and Skye he said to Sabre, "I'm sending those two back to Skye's homeland and I need Misty as well to help with the journey."

"Ah, here you two are. Listen, and if you have any suggestions speak up."

"I need you to go back to Skyes' homeland with an invitation to join us. Tell them about decagon, and that we do have enemies, and explain what we are going to do to rescue our younglings and hopefully, Pearl, my mate. Answer any question honestly, they will know if you are holding out on them. This is where it is important that they do not know you are telepathic, Your shields must be up at all times, otherwise just be yourselves. I know you had a rough flight here Skye, but Misty will help there. We cannot expect all ages of dragons to do that journey in one leg so Misty will raise some islands for them to rest on. But, they either all come or they all stay. That is quite a definite condition, with families and older ones they can show that their intentions are friendly." Rainbow continued, "We have the space and they are welcome. Now, Skye, how many islands do you think the younglings will need so they can rest during the journey? Perhaps you can use the nets for the smaller ones, that would help speed up the trip."

Skye thought for a minute, "I did it in one, but I think they would need at least three stops, the nets will help though>"

"Right," said Rainbow. *Misty, can you come here please?*"he thought.

When Misty arrived, they discussed the journey and what would be needed.

"I can raise three islands if the sea bed is not too deep,there again I've never done it from underwater, hmm, I will give that a test run before we set off. And, we will need fresh water. I also suggest we take a full load of fire chillies, Nothing wrong with being prepared if trouble pops up, and they are rather nice to nibble on and keep your energy up. When they land Meteor and Skye should make out they are exhausted, that way they will; have an edge if it comes to trouble."

"How will we get fresh water to the islands?" asked Meteor.

"Perhaps some of the warriors, they are the strongest and fittest, could take nets full of gushyberries and leave them on the islands, its food, juice and energy in one go," suggested Skye.

His love for gushyberries had not gone unnoticed and everyone laughed!

"That's actually a very good idea, '' said Sabre, "and it still gives us our warrior contingent here. My sea dragons can do that, they can fly out with you, check the sea around where the islands will rise, and warn any life around there to move back to safety, then get back here. Going on what Skye said about the journey, for them I reckon it will take two days at least, once they decide to come. I also suggest that once they are here, Misty if she will, removes all but the central island, eventually we can plant gushyberry trees on it for my dragons to snack on, and maybe some fire chillies as well for the younglings to practise with once we go back to sea."

"We can leave the islands for now; once we get them settled, we can take care of Weld. I know we feel under pressure, but that recipe I read, said it had to be done on a night of the dragon moon, that's over two full moons from now and just before that is a moonless night, that's when we will move against Weld," said Rainbow, "so Misty do you want to go and try underwater island raising?"

Rainbow continue, Sabre, I need you to select your fittest warriors to fly to the islands and back. Meteor and Skye go practice blocking against each other, Peridot can help, she would be delighted to beat you two by getting through. It could save your lives!"

"Emerald, I want you to take Spike to the crystal cave, it's time for him."

"Topaz, I want you to go with Emerald, taking all the other adolescents, ours and the sea dragons. The two of you should be enough. Sabre and I will speak to them before you leave."

"I will do that now if you want me to," said Sabre, "while you get everything sorted."

"Good idea. Thank you Sabre."

Just then, Rae came into the meeting, "What can I do?" she asked.

"I will need you for the battle, but in the meantime, you can help Emerald and Topaz. The goblins have been quiet lately, it won't hurt to have an extra bit of protection, Emerald and Topaz will be going this afternoon, and staying until they have all been through the cave. Thank you Rae."

"Blaze, are you there?" thought Rainbow.

"No! I'm here, Arf! Arf!" she said as she came through the bushes.

"Young Spike is very talented, he is a very good learner as well, and picked control up almost immediately, but I found something interesting. You know you told the younglings to think of ideas.

Well, I'vw come across a very powerful young male, he was invisible and watching Spike and I training, then all of a sudden up he pops and asked to join in properly, he is a little mouse of a thing but very strong in power as a telepath and in invisibility control now he has had the lessons. I've called him Squib for now, as he doesn't want his age group to know. He wants to help search the castle; I think he will be a big help!"

"Oh!" said Rainbow, "but if he is only a youngling it isn't fair to put him in danger is it?"

"Ask him yourself," answered Blaze. "Oy Squib, show yourself; I know you have followed me!"

There in front of Rainbow the air shimmered and there was a little brown dragon who looked at Rainbow defiantly.

"I might be little but I can fight as well as the bigger ones," he said.

Rainbow probed his mind and was shocked to see how he had been bullied by the bigger ones in lessons and in general.

"Why didn't you tell someone?" asked Rainbow.

"I fight my own battles, me and Ice were always being picked on because we are little, so we watched and learned from the warriors, and that's what we are going to be!".

"Well there is nothing like knowing what you want. Is there!" smiled Rainbow, "Go and get something to eat and don't be invisible around warriors again, openly watch and learn. You are now officially an apprentice warrior, and your friend Ice. I want you both back here in one hour, and no mind probing either!"

"That was very nice of you," said Blaze, "how they blocked and hid the bullying, I don't know."

"That needs looking into, and the culprits must be dealt with," said Rainbow Sternly. "Bullying is not what we need in our warriors; I think they may need a stint in Volcano Valley as a lesson. We all depend on each other, whether we are big or small, we are all important and make a difference in each other's lives," continued Rainbow.

"They will learn that up there. Do you think, Blaze, that we should check out all our younglings for hidden powers and talents? They seem to be developing much earlier than they used to, and can be given more responsibilities and trusted more, especially when we are joined by the new dragons. The more eyes and ears the better, as I seriously think they will try and take control here. Power seems to be what they want, just like the bullies, that's why our younglings must be taught better ways!"

"Mentally filling Sabre in on what was happening, he asked for ideas to help the younglings.

I'm on my way back now," said Sabre, *"we'll have a look at our 'New apprentices' and work out a plan of action for them!"*

It was a little while later when two little dragons came before the leaders of the fire dragons, sea dragons and the warriors. They stood their ground steadily and waited for the leaders to speak.

"Right Squib ," said Rainbow, "what is your real name? And, Ice isn't it?"

Ice was a little white dragon who had big blue eyes, and she had a blue tinge to her wings.

"Yes," she said to Rainbow.

Squib looked at Rainbow and said "My real name is awful. Please can I be squib, I like that!"

Thinking about it for a minute, Rainbow said, "If that is what you want, then we will honour your wish, we want no-one unhappy at having a bad name. You are now an apprentice warrior Squib, and you Ice, what are your talents I wonder? Can you tell us, it will go no further."

"Well," said Ice, "I can freeze things with my breath, and I can fly backwards at high speed."

"That's a very handy thing if we need a rearguard. There is a job for you and squib tonight with Blaze. Ice to what degree can you control your freeze? Could you perhaps make it cold so the goblin guards will be more bothered about staying near a fire than patrolling?" asked Rainbow.

"Ooh, yes, that's easy, I did that once to stop the bullies searching for us," replied Ice.

"Right you go with Blaze and she will explain what you are going to do tonight," said Rainbow. "I will tell your guardians that you are on a mission and won't be in tonight. Just remember you are not to be seen or caught. Pearl and the younglings lives depend on that, so keep your wits about you. Go and get some rest now as you will be up all night and I don't want you falling asleep and snoring to give us away!"

Laughing, the two younglings went out to find a quiet spot to sleep.

"What is Squibs' real name then?" asked Sabre, who had been observing the proceedings.

"It's Rat. I would like to know who named him that. It's cruel!"

"Aura, can you give us moment, if you are not too busy," thought Rainbow

As she arrived Aura asked "What can I do for you?"

"We have some younglings here with a problem. I would like you to do some investigating for me please." said Rainbow. "One is small and brown and was named Rat, the other is a white called Ice. They have been bullied. I want to know who named that poor youngling and who has been bullying him and Ice, without them knowing obviously. I don't know who their guardian is but I want you to take over their care please, and if there are any more victims, I want to know who and why it is happening!"

"Poor little mites, of course I will. Where are they?" asked Aura.

"I sent them to get some sleep. They are going out with Blaze to snoop around Welds' castle. Squib has invisibility and Ice has a few talents as well."

"They are not going on their own!" stated Aura, "I am now their defender, and will go as well, and I will not take no for an answer. I am going to talk to Blaze!"

"Well." said Sabre, "you picked a good defender there, and I bet she will know it was that'd behind their problems. There has to be a reason for it."

"You and I," said Rainbow, "come nightfall, will do a flyover Welds' and try to spot all the guards. That will at least show us the clearest way in. I'm holding Peri in reserve, she is a healer now and if anyone is hurt, she will be needed here, and she is also an extra guard for the younglings."

So, they each went off to their allotted tasks and to eat and rest, ready for nightfall.

And so, as the day went on, there were many dragons considering what was to come.. Meteor and Skye were looking forward to their trip. Topaz, Rae and Emerald were in Crystal Valley with their charges. Aura was out and about investigating, and Squib and Ice were fast asleep. . . .

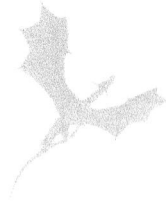

CHAPTER
9

Meteor and Skye were the first to leave, they were to use the moon as a navigational point. They were followed soon after by Misty and the sea dragons, and of course they were all avoiding being seen by unfriendly eyes. Sabre and Rainbow were ready to leave and were just waiting for Aura, Squib and Ice.

Aura arrived first, "I found out what you wanted, Squib and ice were found newly hatched, how they survived I will never know and one of the guards commented that Squib 'looked like a little drowned rat', and, as they were out on patrol for a week the guards looked after the hatchlings. By the time they returned the name had stuck and everyone carried on using it, inconsiderate, but not malicious. Ice was found not far away by the same patrol and she was 'as cold as ice', again the name stuck, especially as she was white and blue. Now as far the bullying goes, there are some culprits. Dawn, Flame and Sapphire. I've got them out with the fishing team for the moment, it will keep them out of the way till we are all back and can sort them! OK!"

"Wonderful job! No wonder they are self sufficient," said Rainbow, "they are coming just now, no word of this for the time being, but they are under my protection from now on, they were obviously part of the stolen clutch."

Ice and Squib were a bit over-awed at first, (and if the truth was known, a bit scared), to be on a mission with Rainbow and Sabre, even Aura was considered a great dragon.

"You two will stay with Aura till we contact you. Can you mind speak?"

"Yes," said ice.

"No" was Squib's reply.

"I will take care of that while you are spying out the land," said Aura, "and remember you two, all our lives depend on you doing exactly as you are told, instantly. Is that understood? This is not a game!"

"Right then," said Sabre, "let's go, and so, by the light of a crescent moon, they took off for the "Dark Side"

Rainbow headed for the coast. "Why are we going to the coastal area?" Ice asked Aura.

"It's simple, you are too small to fly over the ice range, it is cold, high and has very strong winds blowing all the time, the other direction would take too long, so we are going to fly along the coast, just over the sea and avoid being seen. But do keep your eyes open, there may be the odd grawk around. If so, we must destroy them, so they can't raise the alarm, OK?" replied Aura.

It seemed that they had been flying forever, when Aura noticed that Ice and Squib were flaghging. *"Rainbow,"* she thought, *"these two need a rest."*

So Rainbow and Sabre flew underneath the little ones and said "Hold on tight", and piggy backed them so they could rest. So secure were they with their claws locked tight, they fell asleep.

The two. Ice and Squib, woke to the sensation of losing height. Instantly alert they looked around them, but it was dark and the moon wasn't lighting the valley, they could not see much, but knew enough to know they had arrived in the dark side. Ice shivered, and not from cold, which she rarely felt, but a warning tingle.

"There is someone around. I can feel them but I can't see them," she said. Rainbow, Sac

Bre and Aura descended quickly and took cover.

"What can you tell us?" asked Sabre.

"There is one mind, bored and just now and again looking around. I can see through their eyes! It's looking at a courtyard, giggling, and thinking of its dinner. It's a guard, he's very hungry and can't think of anything else. Oh! How horrible, he has just picked up a mouse and swallowed it down."

"Must be a goblin," said Rainbow, "all they can think of is eating. Remember you two, they will eat you as well. Now what are you doing?"

"Shh a minute gob." said Squib, "she is making him do something."

With a look of concentration, Ice slowly started to blow gently, and a thin film of cool air came from her nostrils. Blowing towards what they could now make out as a wall and a faint movement on the top, then it vanished.

Looking pleased with herselfIce turned to them and said "He is cold and hungry, so he has left the wall and gone in through a door on the far side. All he can think of is food and a warm drink. There is no-one else on this side and unless someone else comes out we are clear for now."

"What a wonderful talent," said Aura, "but we need to move quickly while we have the chance!"

Sabre quietly flew up to the top of the wall, being black he was invisible in the dark, and looking round , saw they were at the back of Welds' castle, near what looked like a big garden. Thinking to the others he called them up *That part of the garden is in deep shadow, head for that. I'll keep watch till you are down.*

In a matter of seconds, they were on the far side of the garden hidden behind a hedge, watching and listening, until Sabre joined them. Ice was watching the inner door the goblin had through.

"There is no-one there, but we are being watched. I don't understand."

On full alert, Rainbow said, "Squib, vanish and do a good search around. Sabre can you nip onto the roof area and spy out the land, and Sura, look after ice. I am going back over the wall to check for patrols and look round the other side."

With that Rainbow flew back over the wall and vanished into the dark. Ice hid with Aura behind the hedge, and suddenly, she started giggling quietly.

"Shh, what's wrong?" said Aura.

"It's those two little things, trying to creep up on us, they are funny. I don't think they know I can see them," and mind linking with Aura, she showed what she could see.

"Goodness me, what are they?" said Aura. "Why I do believe that, looking at how that one walked through the tree then, they are ghosts, how unusual!"

As the two hazy shapes drew near, Ice tried to speak to them with her mind, *"Hello, who are you?"*

The reaction was quite funny, they popped in and out of sight three times and clung to each in obvious fear.

"We won't hurt you" said Aura, "can we talk please?"

Slowly, the ghosts calmed down.

"No-one has spoken to us before," said one of the ghosts, "except the white lady and the pink one. All the ugly horrible ones are too stupid to talk to us, and the big mean ones just try and kill us, and they can't, cos, hehehe, we are already killed."

The other ghost continued, "So we help the white lady and the pink girl, they are nice to us, she has got so many children though, it's daft at times. They all jump up and down and flap their wings, it's not as though they can fly, being in dungeons and the doors are shut."

"What are your names?" asked Ice.

"Well I was Beech and he was Elm, we were wood elves till them big ugly ones killed our trees," said Beech.

Elm butted in. "But we get our own back, now we lock doors from the inside and set the rabbits that they eat for free and soak the bed covers. Lots of things we can do."

Aura, having had a warning from Sabre, said, "One of our friends is coming in, he is nice and is called Rainbow. He doesn't like the ugly ones either. We call them agres, and we are dragons. So please don't be scared, or leave. There is another one of us on the roof, he is black and keeping a lookout. Oh, and we have a little one, who can vanish like you, looking around."

Still looking a bit nervous the ghosts went to Ice. "Are you one of us? You are white as well," said Beech.

"I'm a little dragon, so is Squib my friend, and Rainbow, Aura and Sabre look after us," answered Ice.

"I wish we had someone to look after us. The white lady; her and the others are dragons like you," said Beech, "when they take the chains off her she will look after us both. We've been looking through the tunnels for her, so her children can join the pink one and try and get away to her family."

"We are her family," said ice, "we've been searching forever for her and the younglings."

"Younglings! What's them?" asked El,

"Oh, children you call them and Rainbow is like their dad," answered Ice.

Having been warned by Sabre, who had been mind listening, Rainbow slowly approached. "Hello, can \i be your friend too?" he asked.

"Why not," Beech said cheekily, "it's not like you could eat us, ha ha."

The more the wood elves relaxed, the more solid in appearance they became.

"I think we need to have a long talk," said Aura. "Beech and Elm know Pearl and the younglings, and where they are! But we would be wise to move out of here for now."

Turning to the elves, she asked "Is there somewhere we can go that's safe and we won't be seen."

"Yes, with the pink dragon. She will make you happy, she always makes us happy. She is in the closed in garden," said Beech. "I will take you there now, Elm will go ahead and warn her you are coming, she's never had anyone visit her there but us, and will be surprised."

And with a plop! Elm vanished.

Rainbow had been very quiet, to know he had found Pearl and the younglings but couldn't free them broke his heart. But he couldn't think of himself and squashing down his emotions he said, "Lead the way please Beech, Ice tell Squib where we are please and direct him as we go."

So very quietly, with just a murmur of wings they left to meet the pink dragon.

Meanwhile, Squib was having great fun wandering around spying. He'd been in the kitchens and had a few bites out of a delicious big pie, and ran his finger through a trifle, the cream was lovely. Now he was staying out of the way because one of the cooks had found the nibbled food and was ranting and raving about either goblins or ghosts. Thinking it could be fun, he picked up a loaf of bread and floated it to the other side of the kitchen. One of the maids saw it and fainted, fell to the floor and knocked a sack of onions over, they were rolling everywhere causing chaos.

"Squib", came a firm voice in his ear. "You will give us all away messing about like that, Out of there now and meet us in the garden on the opposite side to where we came in. Now!"

Realising he had nearly given himself away, he sneaked to the kitchen door, and found he couldn't open it. He was trapped. Hardly daring to breathe, he sneaked to the door he had come in by, it was a swing door, and the cooks and maids were in and out all the time, getting things from the big pantry next door. So as it swung open he nipped through making sure he didn't touch anyone. Mind you, the tray of buns that was being taken to the pantry was one short when it got there. Just about to enjoy his bun, which he had hidden in his chest pouch, a guard appeared in the corridor. Moving against the wall, Squib stayed out of the way and when the guard said "Send the food down to the prisoners, get the skivvies to do it, I'm not hauling that lot down there, and hurry up."

This was it, thought Squib. He would find the prisoners for Rainbow, and work out how to get them out. He would be a hero. Then no-one would pick on him.

Waiting in the corridor he watched what was going on around him. Eventually a group of miserable goblin prisoners appeared with a large sack over each of their shoulders and trudging to a door at the end went through it.Squib was through it before it had stopped swinging.Sure enough, they came to what looked like cellar steps and just threw the sacks down them.

"I'm not playing maid to any dragon brats, let them help themselves" said one. "If we don't feed the lady one, we will be beaten" said another.

"You go and do it" said another, "We will wait here for you>"

So, the goblin had no choice but to go down the steps.

"How am I supposed to move all these sacks?" he asked as he got further down the stairs.

"One at a time!" laughed the others.

Squib had a problem, all the goblins were at the top of the stairs and he couldn't get past them. Thinking about it for a minute, he went back up the corridor a little bit and took the bun he'd pinched, out of his chest pouch and put it on the floor about a dragon's length away from the goblins. Then sneaking back he thought *"That's my bun, they can't have it"*, and sure enough each of the goblins thought another had said it.

All the heads turned to look, and then, they stampeded after it.

Quick as a flash Squib was down the stairs and by the sacks. Slob, the goblin, was just coming back for another sack, thinking quickly Squib grabbed a sack.

"Oy! What do yer think you are doing?" said Slob.

"The lady sent me to help," said Squib.

"Well, grab two and follow me."

So backwards and forwards they went until nineteen of the twenty sacks were put in a huge vault like a cellar room.

"This should keep you brats quiet for a while," said Slob, "now we will see to the lady."

Dragging the sack Squib followed Slob to a door about halfway down the big vaulted room and unbolted the door.

Squib said to Slob and said, "I'll see to this one if you want."

"Oh yer!" said Slob "and yer will bolt the door again afterwards I suppose, take me for an idiot, go on take her the food and no nonsense."

Squib went forward slowly, dragging the sack, "Good day my lady. I'm Squib if you remember me?"

All the time trying to mind link with the beautiful silvery white dragon lady, chained by the neck and one leg to the wall. Slowly she looked at him, so he did the only thing he could think of, he winked at her! Her eyes opened wide and a distinct look of interest gleamed there.

"Squib, I haven't seen you for a while have I? Who was it you used to play with?"

"Aura, Sabre and Rainbow are my playmates, my lady"

"Oh, I remember them," she said, "how are they, do you still get on well?"

"Yes. We are very close indeed." replied Squib.

"What food have you got me? Can you help me eat as I can't move my neck to reach the food."

"I am not tall enough," said Squib, shrinking into himself. "You'll have to do it," he said to Slob. "Pity there's no key for the neck chain then she could feed herself."

Mind-listening, he caught Slobs' thoughts, the key is on the outside of the door on the wall. The brat could feed her, then she won't eat me. Feeling pleased with his plan he went to the door and got the key.

"If I undo the neck chain lady, you must promise not to eat me," Slob said.

"No, I promise I won't eat you," said Pearl. "You have tried to be nice, and I am very grateful."

So carefully Slob approached the lock on the chain and Pearl looked away at Squib and winked whilst it was unlocked. Then dashing back to the door Slob said to Squib, "Feed the lady and then put the chain back on. When you have finished, bolt the door again", and in a shake of a dragon's tail he was gone.

"That was a very clever move, young dragon, and very brave of you. Please allow me to eat while you tell me what's happening," said Pearl.

Squib told his tale as Pearl ate quickly; she was rather hungry.

She said to Squib, "It's very hard to eat with a chain round your neck, the longer the chain is off the quicker I will be able to mind link with Rainbow. You can mind link, please come here and help me."

Stepping forward, Squib placed his head against Pearls' and called Rainbow.

Rainbow was astounded to hear Pearl calling him, but realised there was not much time to waste on what they really wanted to say.

"I must keep this short, if we can get the chains off, will you be able to walk. How many younglings are with you?"

"Calm down," said Pearl, *"I have been working on a plan for this day. There are things about the castle you need to know, and others here as well."*

Rainbow replied, *"I've met Beech and Elm and we are just about to meet someone called Nattie. Will Squib be safe with you for the moment?"*

"Yes, I can hide him amongst the other younglings", Replied Pearl.

"Good. I will get back to you soon," saisd Rainbow and continued, *"Sabre and his sea dragons ate with us in Secret Valley at the moment, we will soon have you out."*

Right Beech, take us to this Nattie, whoever she is," said Sabre, knowing his brother was in n o frame of mind to plan at the moment. Ice keep up with us and try to keep mind linked with Squib."

Entering a garden with high walls around it, they saw in the shadows a pale dragon who was dancing round a unicorn fountain. It was only as they got closer, in the first blushes of dawn, they could see she was a little beauty and was a lovely shade of pink

She turned to meet them.

"Hello, I am Natalie, but everyone calls me Nattie. I am so glad you have come. Will we all be able to get together soon," she rushed on, "I am a bit fed up not being able to play with the other dragons. I have hundreds of questions for you, but I am being rude. What are your names please?"

"I am Rainbow, Nattie, and Pearl is my mate. I've been searching for since she was captured and the younglings were stolen as eggs. This is Sabre, my brother. This is Aura, one of our family, and this is Ice, and you, Nattie, are one of us!"

With a squeal of delight, Nattie ran to them and spreading her wings gave them all a big hug.

"I have a dragon family at last," Looking at Ice she asked "Are you Pearl's youngling? You look like her."

"You know she's right. And Nattie does too!" said Aura.

"How do you know she looks like Pearl?" asked Rainbow. "I thought you were a prisoner here on your own?"

"Ah" said Nattie, "this is what Pearl wanted me to tell you. You had better get comfy, this will take some time to explain."

With the dragons sitting down in a circle, Nattie began her tale.

"It started when I was very little, not long out of the egg. I have always been pink, but we were all happy together. It didn't matter that we couldn't go out or that Pearl had to wear the chains. We were all together. Then weld started coming down everyday and watched us. Pearl said we were not to show what we could do and to look unhappy and stupid when he was there. Once he had gone, we could all laugh and play. Then one day he stayed a long time and the smallest ones started playing. He did that every day, not moving or saying anything until a lot forgot he was there and took no notice. Then one day he got two eggs that were late hatching and held them over the grate, over the river, which we used as a latrine," she said blushing. "Part of the grid opened but not enough for us to get through. That day Weld asked Pearl what i was but she would not answer. He threatened to break the eggs, but I could not let that happen so I told him I was the happiness dragon, I make everyone feel happy and good. When he heard that, he got angry and threw the two eggs down the grate. I have been sorry ever since, but he would have broken all the other unhatched ones as well. Then, he said to Pearl he was taking me away and then I couldn't make them happy. Unhappy dragons would be easier to control, and if Pearl didn't behave, he would kill me, so she became a chained hostage for our lives."

"It must have been very lonely for you," said Aura.

"It was," continued Nattie, "but then Beech and Elm came to dance and play and it wasn't so bad, they knew where the secret passages were and they would let some of the younglings come out and play with me."

Every so often I would go and see Pearl, and we would talk about what it is to be a dragon. I had lots of lessons with her and the others, while Beech and Elm kept lookout. If anyone was coming, they would go through walls and scare them away.

"It seems my friends that I have a lot to thank you for. I am most grateful to you," said Rainbow. "If you ever want a home with us, you are welcome to be part of our family and we have plenty of beech and Elm trees for you to feel at home in."

"These passages, how big are they?" asked Sabre,"big enough for the younglings to get through?"

"Yes, but not Pearl, she is chained to an outside wall that stands over the river," said Beech. "Is it possible that you can make a hole in it and free her that way?"

"I've been thinking," said Rainbow, "how many can fly, or can't they?"

"Oh yes," said Nattie, "they have been doing wing exercises inside and when they come here, they practice."

"We can get them here and load them into the nets in secret. That will give us a head start on getting them away, and work on the wall without hostages<" said Aura.

"Icen can you help me talk to Pearl," said Rainbow. "Beech and Elm, please can you get Squib out of there, one of the younglings might give him away by asking who he is."

"OK, we will do that now," they both said and with a pop, they were gone.

"I've contacted Squib and Pearl," said Ice, "I can link you directly if you want.

"OK Squib first. Squib there are two ghosts coming to show you the way out, go with them. They are bringing you to us. Do what you can to help Pearl while you are waiting, don't let anyone see you, not even the younglings,"

"OK boss," said quib.

"Pearl, my love, I've missed you. We will be back for you and the younglings, stay brave. We were going to wait for a moonless night but we might as well strike as soon as possible."

While Squib was waiting, he had a thought and tried the neck chain key in Pearl's

leg chains. I worked! Free of the chains Pearl could move around and stretch her wings,

"We will have to be careful no one realises you are free," Squib said.

"Give me a couple of hours out of that iron and I hope my powers will come back" said Pearl, "From now on, we only whisper, so no-one can hear us."

Squib picked up the key from the lock and went out of the cell.

"Back in just a moment," he said. He tried to pick up one of the chains but it was too heavy for him.

"I wanted to take them away from you, so you could recover even quicker!"

!It's all right Squib, as long as it doesn't touch me. If anyone comes, I think we should have the key out of the way. Can you hide it?"

!I will put it in the cell next door, that's where I was going to hide the chains," and moving swiftly Squib slipped out. When he returned, Pearl was still flexing her wings and legs, when 'Pop', in came Beech and Elm.

"Oh, my lady, we are glad to see you are free, and your friends have found you!" exclaimed Beech.

"Shh," said Pearl, "we don't want anyone to know, the first job is to get the younglings free, and then I can fight without worrying."

"Oh, I nearly forgot," said Squib, going into his chest pouch, "Rainbow said you would want these." and he handed over some big fat juicy fire chillies, "will these help?"

"Most certainly." said Pearl, eating them with pleasure.

"Right Squib," said Beech, "you come with us, we will show you a secret way out. I think this is how they want the younglings to get away quietly tomorrow, so watch and learn the way. It might be up to you Squib, to lead the way!", and saying that, Beech led Squib to the end of the cells where there was a big stone wall which had rings in it.

Beech vanished through the wall.

Startled, Squib said, "I can't do that!"

"You don't need to," was Elm's reply, "turn the left hand ring twice, it only goes one way, and then pull it!"

So, Squib did as he was told, and as silent as the night arriving the whole wall swung open.

"This is how you will get out, keep walking forwards, it's a level passage and Beech has the other end open for you. Now pop along and I will close this end."

"How can you close it, when you go through everything?" said Squib. "Ouch!" as his ear was pulled.

"We can do things quite easily when we want," laughed Elm, "how do you think the mustard got in the custard yesterday? And the hedgehogs in Welds' bed, that was great. Shame he ate them though!". And, pulling a lever on the inside wall Elm closed the door up.

Squib walked along the tunnel, unfurling a wing so he could feel how wide it was, it was certainly high enough, and not at all cold and damp. Then he slowly made out a dim light ahead, it was the sky.

Hurrying forward Elm stopped him.

"Always check there is no-one around, 'cept the Pink Dragon, she is a friend."

"Here's the mechanism to open the inside door, and, see this face carved in the outside wall, push the nose in and it opens it from outside. OK it is all clear, your friends are waiting in the shadows over there. Good luck, and we will see you tomorrow night." Elm finished.

And, as quietly as it had opened the door closed.

Keeping a wary lookout, Squib worked his way slowly to the others, he knew you didn't move fast in the shadows or you could be seen, but he went invisible for fun and sneaked up on the others. With them was a pretty pink dragon. Listening for a minute he discovered she was called Nattie and had been a prisoner there as long as the others. Moving round for a better look, Squib found himself pinned to the ground by a huge claw.

"Didn't think you could sneak up like that youngling," said Sabre, releasing him, "You forgot to mind block. Right. It is nearly daylight. Nattie, can you mind link? You can! Great, we are going to vanish for a while and plan for tonight. Get some sleep if you can, it's going to be a long day and night, and we will call you with the mind link at sunset when we are all here.OK!" ended Sabre.

In a flurry of movement, they were gone over the wall and were hidden by the trees. They flew low level till they were out of sight of the castle, and then with Ice and Squib safely in their claws, they set off back to Secret Valley.

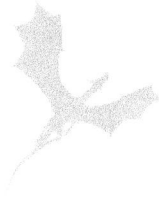

CHAPTER
10

Meanwhile, Meteor and Skye were flying over the sea, Misty and the sea dragons had already created one island, and with Mistys' magic had already got things growing, with a fresh water pool on it. They were flying well ahead of the rest, when, out of the night sky, came a deep screeching noise. It flew towards them in the most threatening manner.

"What is it?" Meteor asked Skye.

"I don't know. I've never seen anything like it!"

Mind linking with Misty they told her what was happening.

"Stay out of its range," replies Misty. *"We will be with you in minutes."*. And she and the sea dragons accelerated to join the two lead dragons.

"I think it is what our teachers called an Atmorphic," said Meteor. "Ohh dragon poop! They are pretty nasty beasts, if it is after us, we must split up in different directions and head back towards Misty and the others. I'm a bit faster than you and can draw it off for a while."

"I can draw it off!" said Skye indignantly.

"Don't you understand that you are the only one who knows where we are going, if need be, the others can take over the mission. I am the expendable one!" said Meteor, keeping an eye on the atmorphic.

It was an outstanding thing, being about the size of a whale. It was something like a cross between a shark and a giant squid, and propelled itself through the air like a jellyfish does in water. As it got closer, Meteor could see the noise was caused by the pulsating body, but he didn't like the look of the teeth and barbs.

"Skye head back to the others now. I can't deal with this if I have to watch out for you as well. Now go, as fast as you can!"

Meteor then turned towards the atmorphic to draw it away from Skye. As he headed towards the creature, he took his fire chillies out and started chewing them.

"Meteor listen, don't look at the atmorphics tentacles, they change colour and have a hypnotic effect, like watching a dancing rainbow. Then, while you are transfixed, they surge forward and get you. Keep your distance, they can move faster than a goblin at teatime!" said one of the sea dragons with Misty.

"Now that is fast", thought Meteor, noticing that the atmorphic had started to weave its tentacles in a pattern. Now there were colours appearing. *"Pretty"* he thought.

An inner warning told him, Meteor move! And, by instinct he flew sideways, just as the atmorphic spurted towards him. It was not fast enough and as they were parallel he fired a burst of flame at it.

Screeching in anger, the atmorphic backed off. Taking stock of this meal that was fighting back! It had never been hurt before, so it started to circle and watch its prey carefully.

Turning at the same speed, Meteor watched carefully. Sure enough, the atmorphic started the colours again but Meteor was ready and gave a huge snort of black smoke and flame making himself invisible to the beast. Stopping down to sea level, but closely watching he mind linked and gave Misty a visual on what was going on.

"Good move, but be careful, they can swim underwater as fast and can fire out of the water at you, get up higher so you have a chance of seeing it," and Misty went on to say, *"some of the sea dragons are in the*

water not far from you. We are approaching out of the sun, be ready to dodge our attack!"

Making sure he was in the clear, Meteor looked around. There was no sign of the atmorphic, it had vanished. Looking downwards, he saw it in the water, but it wasn't hunting him. It had seen one of the sea dragons and was heading for it. Igniting his fire, Meteor dropped as quickly as he could, firing flames at the water, alerting the other dragons, but the atmorphic had him spotted and with a huge water jet propulsion went after Meteor, followed by six sea dragons. With a quick glance towards the sun, Meteor turned and started flying into the light, relieved when he was passed by a swarm of angry dragons, like angry bees they flew down and circled the atmorphic. At the same time as the sea dragons came up from underneath.

"Now" said Misty, and with a giant ball of fire the atmorphic was dragon scorched, leaving just a flutter of ashes dropping into the sea.

"We will make a second island here," said Misty, and asked the sea dragons to check no creatures would be under threat in the area. When she got the all clear, Misty called upon her magic and started the sea bed to rise. The water looked as though it was boiling, and slowly peaks and mounds appeared on the surface. After about an hour, landing on one of the higher hills, Misty said, "I must rest before I generate life and growth here. The sea dragons can swim and feed. Do you want to go with them. You know Skye, you can swim underwater as a sea dragon, and there are some tasty fish down there!"

Stunned at the revelation, Skye wanted to try for himself, to see what being underwater was like, and what fun to chase and catch a fish.

Diving into the water, he soon surfaced, spluttering and coughing, "I thought I could swim underwater?"

"Oops sorry," said Meteor, "I should have told you, you use the same technique for swimming as you do for blocking goblin smell," and demonstrated. "Now try it, you have gills under your scales, and they will breathe for you, relax, enjoy it," and diving back in Meteor and Skye had a jolly good time of it chasing fish and each other.

"Meteor," Misty mind linked, *"can you come up here now please. Oh and a nice fish would be appreciated!"*

So, naturally, they competed as to who could catch the biggest fish for Misty, and surfaced with their gifts. Shaking the water out of their scales they presented them to Misty.

"Sit down and rest," she said. "Thank you for the fish. We must discuss the rest of the journey. Argon the sea dragon team leader tells me we are coming into an area where there are more atmorphics, so I am telling you, for this leg of the journey you will travel with us, and we will fly by night, hopefully avoiding problems. So, get some rest. I have grassed an area over there where you can sleep. I will call you at dusk."

Misty then proceeded to fly to the other side of the island to start work on bringing it to life.

Slowly dozing off Skye said to Meteor, "This is a big island, it should have a name."

"Good idea.W said Meteor.

"We should call it Sea Dragon Island, do you like it?" asked Skye, slowly sinking into dreams of underwater adventures.

Dusk was falling when Misty mind nudged the two sleeping youngsters to wakefulness. Gazing around they were astonished to see the island was beautiful, the growth of grass and trees, even a stream and waterfall. There were even flowers and best of all a large gushyberry tree with fruit on it.

"Misty, this is fantastic; you really are a magical dragon. You must be exhausted",

said Meteor.

"I am a bit tired, so I will rest a while and catch you and the others up later," replied Misty.

"You cannot do that Misty," came the mind thought from Argon, *"Sabre commanded me to stay with you at all times, and I will not put*

you at risk by disobeying a sensible precaution. I have my sea dragons, they will escort these two and I will escort you when you are ready to fly. Accept that or we will all go together."

"*Well that's me told!*" said Misty, "*Very well Argon I will accept your escort most gratefully, thank you.*"

Smiling to herself she explained to \meteor and Skye. Argon and I grew up together, we were always getting into trouble, so Sabre sent me to Rainbow to learn about being a land dragon, so that I could choose my destiny.

The Crystal Cave has already shown me that, now it's up to me to make it happen, and still smiling she lay on the grass and went to sleep, leaving Meteor and Skye to attack the gushyberry tree, which they promptly did and with great relish.

Having explained to Argon the route they were taking, so he and Misty could follow on, and, having eaten all the gushyberries possible, they joined up with the sea dragons and flew off into the dark.

When Misty awoke, she found a big fresh fish and some gushyberries by her,

"I thought you might be hungry," said Argon. Get something inside you, and then we can start out before it gets too light."

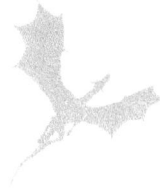

CHAPTER
11

In the Crystal Valley, Rae, Emerald and Topaz were supervising the young dragons and Spike was trying to help by overflying the valley on lookout duty.

All was going well; the young ones were going into "The Cave of Destiny, and coming out as adults. The sea dragons were seriously in awe of the caves' beauty and magic. The land dragons were more familiar with what it was all about, and assumed a nonchalance that made them look wiser than they were. Some had changed colour, some had grown,and each one as they went through their time in the cave had changed.

Whilst he was overflying the river Spike spitted movement between the river and the trees, dropping below the skyline so he wasn't seen, he made a second pass, sure enough the goblins were there, setting up camp. About thirty of them.

"Whoops trouble" he thought to Topaz, *"About thirty of them, by the river, everyone get out of sight."*

"Stay out of sight yourself," replied Topaz, *"Rae and Emerald will be with you soon."*

"Oh goody! A bit of fun" came the mind thought, as Blaze flew down and joined them.

"They have used that site before, never learn do they! Mmm I bet the young sea dragons have never seen any crispy goblins before, shall we go and get a "Take away" ladies, and tidy up a bit. Arf Arf!"

Flying low the three dragons headed for the river, keeping a vigilant lookout for straying goblins.

"There's one in that clearing," said Blaze.

"I'll get it!" said Emerald swooping down and crispy frying the goblin.

"Any more while I am down here?" she asked, and spotting a movement in the corner of her eye she turned a beam of fire onto the bushes. Going forward to investigate, she found another goblin. . . roasted!

"Think you have cleared that area, they are obviously working in pairs, and must be a bit nervous, hee hee," said Rae from above. *"Spike, we are near the bend in the river, where are you?"*

"I am swimming up the river towards you, the goblins were getting a bit close so I popped into the water and submerged," came the reply, *"They have about four patrols in pairs out at the moment!"*

Blaze, showing remarkable agility for a dragon of her magnificence, suddenly pounced, like an owl on a mouse, and came up with yet another goblin.

"There must be another one around here if they are in twos", she said.

Just then, with a lot of splashing and a flurry of dragon wings Spike appeared with a very wet goblin in his jaws. "They taste quite good fresh as well", he said. "Want some?" offering bis goblin.

"No thanks," said Rae, "We've got one each. I suggest we hide them in the bushes until we've sorted the other ones out, then the rest can join us for a picnic. That will sort supper out."

Now, when a dragon wants to be stealthy, they are remarkably light footed and can somehow slip through bushes with comparative ease. Moving forward slowly, they got in range of the goblins camp and studied it carefully.

"*You know,*" thought Blaze, "*we could bring the young ones who have done the cave and give them some training, shall I summon them?*"

"*What a good idea. Tell them all to fly low and we will meet them by the river upstream. See what plans they come up with!*" thought Rae.

And so, a great adventure for the young ones was set in motion. Topaz rounded up all the young adults and explained the situation to them.

"There are still some to enter the cave, I think we should all go and finish the destiny after. Or do you want the cave first? Either way is right, you that have changed could go as a group and we will join you in a couple of hours. What do you want to do? Go and talk amongst yourselves and decide."

The six came back and asked Topaz, "Could we all go into the cave together? Then there won't be much delay,it would be a shame if we died not knowing what our destiny is, and, perhaps we will have a skill that may be useful."

"Let me check," and going into the cave Topaz spoke, "Spirit of Destiny, you know what is in my mind, can you do this?" Topaz was sure she heard a chuckle.

"Your dragons that came to me originally, were sheltering in the cave from meteorites, about fifty of them, so as they needed guidance, I made myself known, so bring in your few and we will not have any problems."

Mind calling the six, Topaz said, "*Go in and do what you are told. Each one of you will be mind linked separately to the Spirit of Destiny. Good luck and enjoy the experience.*"

Next, she had to join the others, who she was glad to see had organised fire chillies, and made them into packs for their chest pouches, and she was pleased to see seven spares. They had thought of her and the six. A good sign.

"Right1, said Topaz, looking at the,. "You the large gold, what is your name please?"

"Sol," the gold dragon answered.

"OK," continued Topaz, "you are in charge until you meet up with Blaze, Emerald and Rae. I want you to head out at low level towards the pinnacle on the other side of the valley and then fly carefully down river, using what cover you can. Sol, if you see any goblins you must deal with them quickly and quietly. Emerald tells me they are in pairs, so if you only see one you had better search for its partner so it can't alert the others. I'm relying on you Sol! Take good care, and mind link if you need help. An open call will do it."

"Now, what's next?"

Topaz headed back to the cave entrance and sat inside, just out of sight of anything walking or flying past. Waiting for the last six to find their destinies, not that anyone discussed it. It was a dragon's private secret, and only they knew. Which gifts they had was ok to talk about, but anything else was taboo.

Further along the valley Blaze and the others were vigilant. Waiting for the group to arrive, they had just settled down when a shout was heard from down river.

"Scabby, Belcher, are you around?"

"Hey-ho," said Blaze, "more gobble ups. Hide in the bushes around the clearing on that side and I will wait here and have a nap, you know what to do." she said with a wicked grin.And so, it was that searching for Scabby and Belcher, two more goblins turned up.

"Oy, what's that?", asked one of the goblins looking at the reclining figure on the other side of the clearing.

"Shh. It's A dragon!" was the answer

"And, she was trying to sleep," said Blaze.

"Ohh, good grief it's talking!"

"Correct," said Blaze, opening an eye and staring at them. What are you apart from ugly?"

"We are goblins," said the one hiding behind his friend. "Ain't you ever seen one before?"

"Oh yes," said Blaze, "including your two friends, if you look over there behind that big bush, they are lying down."

So they went toward the bushes, and were obliterated by a wall of fire.

"And now there are four, at this rate there won't be any left for the others to deal with," said Blaze. And she promptly closed her eyes and went to sleep.

While the young dragons were heading off into their first battle action , trying to look serious, but bursting with excitement really, Topaz waited patiently inside the cave, until she heard quiet talking and footsteps. Peering outside, she saw two goblins, discussing if there were any wild animals in the cave, and if it would be a good place to have a couple of hours sleep.

Slowly moving further back into the darker side of the cave, using her mind link, she warned the "Spirit of Destiny" who told her this was nothing to worry about. The cave protected itself, and promptly a dozen large snakes appeared on the floor, writhing and hissing towards the cave entrance, where they stayed as guards. The goblins heard the hissing and started to back away slowly, and when they were far enough away, they turned and ran at great speed, as far away from the cave and its scary denizens, and didn't stop till they had crossed the river.

It was a good while later when the first of the six came out of the "Destiny Grotto" and the transformation was spectacular; she was a wonderful Blue and was a bit stunned by it all. Next came a handsome Bronze male, with eyes as green as emeralds, One by one, they came out, astonished by their change, and at the others, there was only one left so Topaz went to look for him, he was hiding and weeping.

"Why, what on earth is the matter?" asked Topaz.

And , a forlorn grey looked out of tearful eyes and said, "The others are magnificent and look at me! I'm just Grey."

"Don1t be silly." said Topaz, "We never know what greys are going to be straight away, it takes a while for your colour to develop.

Rainbow and Sabre were grey to start off and look at them. What's your name, for now, anyway?"

"Were they really! I'm Rock."

"I don't tell lies young dragon, come along now the others are waiting. You will find your destiny soon, don't worry about that!"

When they all emerged into the sunlight, they all looked at each other's scales glinting in the sunlight; even Rock had a sheen on him.

"Come on. Let's go after the others. Rock you scout ahead and watch out for those goblins. We will be right behind you." said Topaz.

And so, they took off looking for adventure and their fellow dragons. The first group reached the pinnacle with no problems, it was as they approached it, they saw movement and sure enough there were two goblins on watch. Sol put on a burst of speed and cut them off.

"Quick, push the rocks down and stay below the skyline, W and pouncing on the petrified goblins Sol put them out of their misery with one snap of his mighty jaws. The falling rock hid them from sight.

"With a bit of luck, they will think it is a landslip. A sad accident. Let's get undercover down by the river and I will call Blaze and the others."

"When Sol mentally called it was Rae who answered, *Follow the river carefully so that you are not seen. We will meet up with you in the first big clearing on the left bank.*"

Within a few minutes the two dragons had met up, and were sharing information. The older dragons were quite impressed at the way the young ones had dealt with the pinnacle dragons.

"Good thinking Sol," said Blaze, "how do you fancy being a warrior, we have a need for quick-thinking dragons. Think about it."

"Whilst everyone was wondering what they could do Emerald came forward and said, "I need a few of you to help me please. When the others join us, they will be bound to be hungry, as will you. I know a very good place with lots of rabbits, all quite plump, shall we go and get some? We could put them on a slow cook over the fire pit, and that's the meal sorted, ready for after. They will go nicely with crispy goblins. Nothing like a good meal after a goblin hunt!"

"When they all returned, Blaze called to them. "The other group is coming into range, they will be here very quickly, and then we have to work out a plan of attack. Remember, these are goblins, nasty, vile creatures who think nothing of boiling a dragon egg, or eating a youngling if they catch one. We will protect our own, and future generations, so don't hesitate. Every one of them we wipe out is one less for Weld to control or defend his castle. We are going to join Rainbow and Sabre in a rescue mission, some of you will be in the attack line and some of you will handle rescue nets. Each one of you will do the task you are assigned without any argument. We will have absolute dragon obedience on this; our very future depends on this."

When the other group arrived, the younger dragons were happy to chat about their changes in size and colours, all but Rock, who kept to one side.

"Hmm" said Rae, after welcoming topaz back to the group, "What's wrong with the young grey?"

"He thinks he is a failure because he is grey and plain," replied Topaz.

"I know just the thing to help him," said Blaze, "just give me a few minutes to talk to Rainbow."

"We mind linked and I could see Welds' castle and surroundings, he will mind link when we all get together, and you can all see his plan in one go."

After about five minutes Blaze said, "Right we have got a plan. What's the greys' name?"

"Rock, can you come here please, we have a mission for you" was the first open mind call.

Looking surprised Rock headed towards the group of elder dragons, whilst all the young ones looked on with envy. Seeing this made Rock feel very important, and he hurried to them.

"How can I help you, my lady?" he asked Blaze.

"Well first thing is, you call us by our names, you are an adult now and our equal. Secondly, I know you feel left out by being grey, but it is the greatest thing that could happen for now. We need a dragon that can be camouflaged against the grey granite walls of Welds' castle as a spotter once the mission is underway. You can almost be invisible against the turrets, and from up there you can tell us what is happening in the different courtyards, can you do this?"

"I know I can, who would I relay the information to?"

"Me." said Blaze, "I will be your relay to the others, that way the mind speak won't get cluttered up with open links, but first of all I need you to get up onto that cliff face over there and not be seen. Then spread your wings a little to break up your shape, and watch the goblins camp for me, they should all return there soon for their evening meal. I need to know when they are all settled and relaxed. So, grab yourself a rabbit to eat and rest for a little while, and if the others want to know what you are going to do, don't tell them! We will keep them guessing. I can't have other dragons knowing about my undercover spy, can I? Arf! Arf!"

"Rae, can you show Rock how to break up his shape and a few other camouflage tricks as you show him where the best observation point will be, and after that, it is on you Rock."

The attack happened just a s planned, they waited until all the goblins had gathered and then they destroyed them

With a quick efficient barrage of flames, the sort only a flight of dragons could achieve.

"It was quick and clean, more than they deserved," said Emerald, "Oh look!" and there on the rocky cliff face was a giant blast of fire. "Good chap that Rock; he found a couple of strays and has dealt with them, that's initiative for you!"

"Yes," said Blaze, proud of her protege, "you all did a wonderful job, you really are "Dragons!"

It was as a heron Rock was welcomed back into the group.

"What happened?" Rae asked.

"It was just as the wall of flame started, I saw two goblins that were just coming back, they were arguing about some snakes in a cave. When they saw the flames they ran for cover, and started up the cliff, like ants they were and so I waited till they came into range and shouted, they stopped dead with surprise and I zapped them!"

"What did you say?" asked Topaz.

Looking a bit sheepish, Rock said "Boo!"

This set the whole group laughing, and the dragons were in good spirits.

"Let them enjoy it while they can, Rainbow has been in touch. We are to fly directly to the Dark Side, I have the rendezvous points. There will be fire chillies waiting, we are going in very soon to rescue Pearl and the younglings." said Blaze.

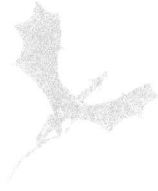

CHAPTER
12

While Misty was resting, the rest of the group set off on the next leg of the trip.

"How on earth did you manage it in one flight?" asked Meteor.

"Well," said Skye, I knew that the winds higher up were stronger and blew in the right direction. So, I went up and used my wings to glide a lot, that was quicker and saved strength, but coming from this direction, the wind is against us. That's why we are creating the islands, then even if the wind veers round, everyone will be able to do the trip."

"No-one will be left behind for any reason," said Meteor.

"I am beginning to wonder if we will need three islands, we've done quite well so far," mused Skye.

"Don't forget," said Meteor, "there will be younglings and the elderly and inferm. We are fit; some of them may need nets to help them, and the quicker we are,the sooner we can get back and help Rainbow. I shall be glad to be with him."

Misty was already on her way to join the rest, accompanied by Argon, They flew swiftly to join the others and located the position of the next island to be made.

"Skye, how far inland are your clan? Have they been to the coastal region?

"I flew for about a quarter of a morning before I was over water. The elders told me to look for a mountain shaped in a point, and that was the direction I had to fly. Someone must have been that way! How else would they know? And why couldn't we have lived by the sea? There's a lot I don't understand! Were the Elders desperate to keep power over us? I was always asking questions. Meteor, do you think, the elders sent me on this mission hoping that I would fail and die? Why?. What are they afraid of?"

"I don't know," replied Meteor, "they are your clan. Were the Elders that bad?"

"Yes! Having lived with your dragons," answered Skye, "we wereno better than slaves, doing whateveer they wanted. You are all free, and work together for the good of each other. Look there's the top of an underwater mountain sticking up. This could be a good place for the next island, we can leave the sea dragons to tell Misty while we carry on."

"We need to let her know which way we went though, she is following us in. Will you tell one of the others? I'm just going for a fish, I am starving."

And with that Meteor plummeted into the water looking for a nice fat fish, followed a little while later by Skye and the other dragons. It was feeding time.

"This is what I mean," thought Skye. *"Why haven't we been living like this, eating fish instead of going hungry? The younglings are stunted in their growth through lack of good food. Why do that to yourself, when it can be prevented. Look how I have grown since you found me!"*

Meteor thought for a while. *"If it is power they want, then perhaps keeping everyone smaller and weaker is the way they are doing it, but why? That puzzles me."*

Having eaten their fill, they climbed onto the rocks jutting out of the sea to dry their wings in the sun. Keeping a wary eye out for atmorphics and other threats. They were soon ready for the off.

"One thing," said Meteor, "We Don't know how far out our mind links will transmit, so can you all shield your minds, and we will only talk from now on. OK?"

And like a pair of winged avengers, Skye and Meteor launched themselves into the air and vanished into the distance. The sea dragons were getting the area ready for Mistys' arrival and her terraforming magic.

Flying at a great height, it wasn't long before they saw the distant shorelines and a great pointed mountain on the edge. Veering towards it, they reinforced their mental blocks and flew to the rapidly approaching land mass.

At first they were buffeted by warm air and winds coming off the ground, then slowly adjusted their flight, headed the way Skye indicated, towards the unknown family of dragons, and an even more unknown welcome! The land beneath them was almost desert scrub land, and monotonous.

"How on destinys' whim did you put up with such a miserable area?" asked Meteor.

"Until I flew over the sea, I knew nothing else, '' was Skye's answer. "We've made good time, I think,we should land for a minute while we are alone and can talk."

Landing, Meteor could see his friend was troubled.

"If I was sent off to be gotten rid of. I don't know what sort of welcome we will get, so don't trust, and watch for mind probes. I'm going to call you Lord Meteor,if they think you have status, they may be careful how they treat you, and I was going to suggest we keep quiet about \misty and Argon joining us later. What do you think?"

"That could be a good move, until we know more about how they will react, I will act as though it is a rescue mission and we've come to save them! HE he, Lord Meteor, I like that!"

Having decided on a tough plan of action they launched into the sky and headed towards Skyes old home. It was a bit of a let down really, when they got to their destination a large sandstone cliff with hundreds of caves in it, and the area was dull and brown. Nothing like the lush green areas of decagon, and the air was so arid and dry. Coming into land there was no trace of anyone around.

"Where is everyone?" wondered Meteor out loud.

"Oh, they don't have lookouts and always hide till they see who it is." said Skye.

Sitting down to wait,it was not long before a number of dragons emerged from one of the larger caves and moved slowly forward. Skye went forward to them, slowly followed by Meteor.

"Elders I wish to make known Lord Meteor, ambassador from the King of the Dragons of Decagon. He is here to offer you a new home,and the land is rich and fertile. Trees, water,everything we need. My lord, the elders of our Dragons."

One dragon in particular stepped forward and looked at Meteor, "But you are a mere youngling!"

"With the greatest respect to your age, I am the senior warrior after our second in command Lady Blaze, and , I have been tasked by Rainbow our King to see what assistance you need,and to offer you a home on decagon, where you will be welcomed as long lost relatives. It will be me you deal with and I have the power to act accordingly. We have come in friendship, but I will take no insult from you or any other Elder who maligns my badge of office."

And doing so, he reached into his chest pouch and brought out a magnificent jewel on a chain of gold and put it over his head. "This is the eternal stone, one of the jewels of King Rainbow and it gives me authority to negotiate, or to return home!"

Astounded at the sight of the jewel the first Elder reached forward to grab it, but Meteor was not a senior warrior for nothing. His talons expanded and his arm swept towards the Elder, stopping just short of his throat.

"Skye, name these Elders for me so I know with whom I am dealing please."

"Pah! You tell them, you don't indulge them. My name is Norgra. I am the leader here, and they do as they are told!" He said glancing around at the other dragons that had slowly come out of the caves.

"Really, we have no need to bully our dragons. '' said Meteor, "and please and thank you are just manners to us, nothing namby pamby about it, we ask, and the results are happy dragons who trust us. Still different ways, different clans, I am sure when you have your "Dragon Roar" and talk to yours they will be happy to travel to a new home. We have space, and we even have valleys full of herds to feed everyone, and I am sure they will love the gushyberries, especially the younglings."

"Are you ready Skye? We will go and set up camp over there I think, give these good dragons the chance to get over the surprise of your return from a successful mission. I am sure you will excuse us Elders and Norgra, while we let you talk things over."

"Do you have family here Skye? You will probably want to go to them," Meteor asked as they went to set up camp.

"My father went missing a few months ago and my mother and sister are still here. I will go and see them now, and warn them to be ready to leave at short notice. They are coming to Decagon. As the only family male, it is now my duty to protect them," was Skye's answer.

"Oh, if Norgra tries to question you, tell him how good it is, but don't let him bully you, you are one of us now, and don't mind link, we will keep that our secret till everyone is safe on the mountain and Norgra can't interfere. Go see your family, I will come and see them in a while.."

Sitting down after setting up camp, Meteor looked around him, these dragons were in a sorry state, only the elders looked well fed, and, the rockpool that supplied the water was guarded, but the elders went and drank when they wanted. None of the other dragons would look at them, even when spoken to.

"Seems to me they need shaking up a bit round here Meteor thought to himself. Rising majestically, Meteor went to the water pool for a drink, he was followed at a distance by four younglings. As he approached the guard stepped forward and said, "I'm sorry, this pool is off limits to all but the Elders, you have to use the small one round the back of the rocks over there."

Drawing himself to his full height and letting his barbs and talons show, Meteor said in a very loud voice, which carried a fair way.

"You are breaking one of the sacrosanct laws of Dragonkind. No-one is denied water amongst our race by the will of our God Draco. Who are you to deny me the right to life-giving water?"

And, as his voice echoed around the camp a second voice joined him, "By all that is sacred to Dragons, who gave this order?"

And seemingly from nowhere Misty in all her glory appeared. "Well I am waiting for an answer?"

A very timid voice said "Leader Norgra your majesty," and at that a very angry Misty called "Norgra come here and answer to me!"

Hurrying to see what the commotion was Norgra and the other Elders came forward.

"Who are you to summon me like a dog?" growled Norgra.

Meteor stepped forward, "May I introduce Princess Misty, heir to King Sabre, and this warrior is Lord Argon," indicating yet another ferocious looking warrior dragon. "He is the Princesses champion and bodyguard."

"Enough of the introductions, I want to know why this pool is guarded? Against all the Dragon laws this is the most serious crime against your own dragons. Explain yourself!" demanded Misty

"This is Norgra my lady and it is on his instructions the pool is closed to all but the Elders," said Skye stepping forward.

Norgra realising he was in deep dragon poop and bowed and explained,"We have to conserve the water, we can1t have the younglings playing with it can we?"

And with a smile he thought he was charming Misty, but it got him nowhere.

"Where is your water source, is it up in those mountains?" said Misty, pointing to a distant mountain range. "I wonder If there has been a rockfall, or something that is slowing the water down"

Norgra and all the others looked at each other in alarm, then blanked their expressions, but not before Misty and Argon had seen the looks.

"Perhaps my lady, when you have rested , we could fly over there and investigate," suggested Argon

"There's nothing over there, We went and looked; it's an underground stream that is not easy to get to as there is only one place where it comes to the surface. It's not worth wasting your time with. Now that range on your left is much nicer to look at. There are a couple of valleys with trees in them, very pleasant in this heat," concluded Norgra.

"Well, why are your own dragons not there, instead of this barren land. What sort of leaders are you? Where are your families? Are they here or are they there?

These questions were making the Elders very nervous, and they were edging away from Misty and Argon.

"Right, that can wait for now, this water business wants sorting. I am sure it was over caution on your part, but since we are here to take you all back to Decagon, there is no problem,. Do you want to tell your families to return for departure, because there is no way we can leave you to live like this! Would you like that younglings? Woodlands and meadows, lakes and streams we even have an ice valley and snow on some mountains you can play in."

"But what about our work?" asked one youngling.

"What work?" asked Meteor puzzled.

"That's enough younglings!" interrupted Norgra, "Why not go home now."

"Just a minute" Come here young one," said Misty gently. "What work do you do, please tell em."

"We have to dig the earth on the other side of those rocks and sift out any of those white pebbles and the yellow stones for the Elders," said the little one.

"Can you show me what you do?"

"Oh, we all do it, our parents included, that's how we earn our food now!"

Skye and Meteor had been watching and they saw Norgra and the others gathering. Slowly lowering his mind block he listened as they discussed what to do. It had paid off keeping their telepathy a secret. Now they knew what the enemy, and they were enemies, were plotting against them.

"I am going back to the camp in a minute," said Meteor, "do you want to put your stuff with ours Argon, before your investigation?"

Looking straight at Argon and Misty he made eye contact.

"That's a good idea; we can freshen up while the younglings tell their parents where they are going."

"Yes! What a good idea," said Norgra, " but I am sure you will soon see that it is a game the younglings have made up! Why don't we all meet up back here in a short while, we will wait here for you."

Once out of earshot, Meteor explained that the elders are going to group together and mind control the other dragons, to make out it was a younglings game. The other alternative was to kill them in the valleys and make out it was a landslide.

"What are they hiding, and why make their own dtragonsmind slaves," wondered Argon.

It was a puzzled Skye who said, "I don't understand. When my father was leader we had plenty of food and water and no-one was a slave, oh and these are the pebbles and rocks they want, my sister had some in her pouch."

"Misty looked and laughed. "This explains a lot. Watch!" and using her power rubbed the pebbles in her claws; they were transformed into beautiful jewels and the rocks into gold dust. "There is a legend that once our race was obsessed with treasure of any sort. Well we have evolved past that, but sometimes you get odd ones that show that tendency. They are dragon hoarders. Have you ever seen where they sleep, Skye?"

"No-one is allowed into their caves."

"That's because they are using treasure as their beds. They love to lie in gold and jewels; personally, I can't see the pleasure of lying on lumpy old stones."

"So, that s what my father meant!" Skye exclaimed. "He said that this was the worst place for dragons to live, and we must move to the valleys if we can find a main water source there, or find a new home completely as this place would destroy us!"

"Well he was obviously a wise dragon; he knew that the very presence of this lot would slowly corrupt some of you. It is a good job you are all coming with us to decagon. Our problem is to get Norgra and his cronies to leave this treasure behind" said Misty.

"I think if they caused any objections, we will just leave them here and in a couple of moon passes we can message them and see if they have changed their minds"

"There is nothing like a bit of hardship, and doing your own work to make you think again. The other sea dragons will be here today to help move the weak and the young ones. I just hope it goes smoothly or we may have to use a dragon roar to shock them and to let them know we are more powerful and intelligent than they think. Now Argon and I are going to explore, they can think we are going to look at the valleys, but I have a strong feeling we need to look at the range they don't want us to."

"Meteor, I want you and Skye to fly towards the sea and intercept the sea dragons, tell them what's going on and to be just ordinary dragons and mind block. We will be back later on."

So with plans made the four dragons went to where Norgra and the other elders were waiting. "Let's go talk to those younglings then.

When they went behind the rocky outcrop, they saw a small pool of water in the rocks, nowhere near as much or as clean as the 'Elders pool'. And joined all the dragons young and old.

Nogra jumped in straight away, "The younglings have been making a tale up of them digging, I have explained that it is just a game but can you all reassure our guests, that, that is all it is, 'A game'."

And using telepathy he ordered them all to agree, but somehow it didn't work.

One of the mothers said, "A game! Is that what you call it? We have been working here for you for at least two moon falls, and I am sick of the dirt. My talons are ruined and you make the younglings do it as well. And we have no idea why. Oh I know you control the water so we have to do as you say."

As all the others started complaining as well, Norgra and his cronies beat a hasty retreat to their caves.

"Argon can you explain to them what has been happening" said Misty, "Ijust want to go check these rocks out>"

So, while Argon told them about the mind control and what they had been digging, Misty walked to the rocks she was interested in. Placing her claws onto the rock, she concentrated.

"What is it?" asked Meteor who had followed her.

"There is an underground stream, but it is partly blocked, and not naturally either. Everyone stand back, I am going to release it/"

And summoning her powers she cleared the blockage, and slowly you could hear a distant gurgle.

"We will need a pool for it to go into as well."

Slowly the rocks sank into the ground leaving a big rocky hole that was ready, and with a great roar all the blocked-up water flowed into the pool.

"Now the blockage has gone the water will trickle in steadily, so now you have fresh drinking water on the other side, and, well I guess this could be a large pool for bathing and playing in. What do you think younglings?"

And without ado the dragons all jumped in, mums washing the younglings, dads were playing with them and before you knew it, they were all lovely shiny dragons again, shimmering in the sunlight.

So, all being amicable, Meteor and Skye set off to meet up with the sea dragons, and Aragon and \misty set off in the direction of the mountains. Once they were out of sight though, they veered off to the other range of mountains and started to search from above.

"Just what are we looking for, my Lady?" asked Aragon.

"I'm not sure, but I have seen this range before in the Cave of Destiny. So, I know there is something I must do here. What? I am not sure, but I feel something drawing me on. Let's go over there it looks familiar."

So, they headed down a canyon towards a rock face with caves in it.

"Lets search these. Whatever is calling to me is here somewhere," said Misty.

"Don't you think we should mind sweep to see if anything nasty is in them?" said Argon, "don't want to disturb a grawk nest or anything nasty do we?"

In the first few caves, there was nothing except the odd snake or two, but as they got nearer to the biggest cave of all, they picked up a thought. It was just a wave of pain, but it was a conscious mind that made it.

"Hello, can you hear me?"

"Do you need help?"

The thought that came back was *"I am finally going mad. Draco spare me insanity."*

"You are not insane, we are outside the cave, is it safe to enter and help you?"

"There is a big pit between me and the entrance. That's all I know. Who are you? And how can you mind speak?"

"We are dragons, I am Misty and Argon is with me. Who are you?"

"So am I, my name is Pulsar. please help me get out of here. My son is in danger and the rest of my clan. I must get to them and warn them."

"We are coming in, and I'm going to use fire to see where this big hole is, so don't be afraid"

Advancing carefully, Misty let out a small flame, enough to see by. They soon found the big pit.

"If he is badly hurt, we can't get him out easily. Pulsar there will be some shaking and noise so do not be alarmed, just trust us."

And just like that Misty closed the pit up, the ground trembled a bit and a few rocks fell. But Misty had it down to a fine art and everything settled quickly. Moving on guided by Misty's flame, they came to a bend in the cave, and just around the corner was a dragon. He was fastened to the rocks with an iron chain.

"Who has done this to you?" and MIsty used her fine control of fire to make a needle beam of flame and melted the shackles, which Argon kicked away from them.

Using her power, Misty tapped into the rock and a slow trickle of water came forth. Pulsar drank and drank and with the release from the shackles and the water he seemed to visibly improve.

"I couldn't do anything with those on, thank you, you have saved my life."

"I think the sooner we are out of here the better," said Argon, "let's go to one of the other lighter caves and see what damage is done to you. Can you walk?"

"I'm a bit wobbly, but I think I can. I don't know about flying though."

"Let's just get to the cave mouth and check outside first!"

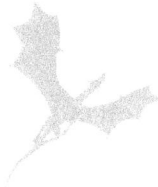

CHAPTER
13

S lowly, with one on each side of him, Pulsar moved towards the cave entrance. "Where did tht pit go? I know it was there!"

Argon just chuckled. "Misty thought it was dangerous so she closed it. It has made it easier for you to get out, hasn't it?"

And with Pulsar still wondering , they reached the cave mouth.

"Wait here," said Argon, "I am going to check around first."

Using his telepathy like sonar he caught a very faint ping, quite some distance away but approaching.

"We must move out of here quickly. Down there is a cave at the bottom of the chasm. Can you glide down there if we help you?"

Pulsar flexed his wings and said, "Let's go then."

Soon they were gliding down to the bottom and a cave that was very hard to spot. Pulsars' landing was a bit wobbly but he was down safely, and they entered the cave. Argon didn't dare use his sonar again in case whoever it was felt the pulse.

"Misty, can you make that cave entrance fall? If they think that Pulsat has been killed in a rockfall, whoever it is might just go away?"

Argon opened his chest pouch and said to Pulsar, "Here eat a few of these, might help. These are fire chillies, but jolly good to eat, give you some energy and Ha ha, some fire in your belly."

"Fire chillies? I didn't think they really existed, and do they.... er... well!"

"Yes," said Misty putting him out of his embarrassment, "we can produce fire, and they are a good food source. How have you heard of them?"

"Just in stories, passed down. I thought that's all they were just stories."

"How about you tell us how you got into that cave and who is in danger? We can help," said Misty.

"It's all right, I'm keeping watch," Argon reassured Pulsar.

"Well, I don't know how long I've been in there, but I was the leader of a group of dragons. We had to leave our home because all the water dried up, so we came to this area and set up a temporary camp, while we explored the area for a new home. But, some of our group found jewels and gold and got the ancient treasure hoarding compulsion. I tried to stop them, but they threw iron chains around me. They flew me here dangling from the chains, as helpless as a youngling in its shell. They must have planned it because they had food and water in the cave on the other side of the pit. They hauled me over in the chains and fastened them to a rock. I tried to make the food and water last, but it ran out. The weaker I got the more the iron burned me, I'm sure the chains were enchanted. The pain was awful if I tried to think of escape. Now they have taken over my dragons and I couldn't do anything to stop them. It's my son, he was to be the next leader and they will no doubt try to get rid of him in some way. Make it look like an accident!"

Misty was smiling as she said, "Don't worry, Skye is alright and your people are as well. Skye was sent across the sea to find a new land, and he found us, the dragons of Decagon and our leader Rainbow, and the sea dragons who have Sabre as their leader. Rainbow has sent us to collect all dragons and to return you to a new life in Decagon, where you will never want again. No-one has treasure fever and we have space enough for everyone. You will have your own valley and still lead your people, and once you have done the Cave of Destiny, like \Skye, you will know what is foretold for you. Skye is one of our warriors now, by his own choice and has become a great adult, well respected; you will see a big change in him. He will be back in camp with his mother and sister, awaiting some more of our dragons here to help you back to Decagon.

Slumping down with relief, Pulsar was overcome with emotion.

"By the star of Draco. The thoughts I had nearly drove me crazy. That Skye would be killed, and my wife Cloud and daughter Star would be prisoners at Norgras' mercy, especially as breeding females."

"Right, do you feel well enough to start out towards the others? Said Misty, "we need to keep you hidden for now, until you regain your full strength, and that means eating! I think we have time to hunt for a few rabbits and eat, don't you Argon?"

"I'll go and find something," Argon volunteered, and flew off to hunt, keeping a wary eye out.

It wasn't long before he returned with a rather plump Reedonk. It was like a cross between a rabbit and a small cow, and a very welcome meal it was too.

Pulsar sighed with contentment, he could feel the strength slowly returning to his limbs and before he knew it he was fast asleep. Leaving him to rest, Argon and Misty went to the cave entrance and watched from the cave shadows.

"Think they are still here?" asked Misty, "whoever it is! I think Norgra thinks we're stupid and we won't think one of his councils will come to check that Pulsar is still locked up, the rockfall will deal with that hopefully."

"I've been thinking," said Argon, "Pulsar can't rejoin his dragons yet, but we could take him to the coast and he can swim and fish till we are all heading over there, and he can be hidden amongst the sea dragons. What do you think?"

"I can't swim ," said Pulsar. Laughing Argon told him all dragons and swim and breathe underwater.

"We will show you, it's the best way, you can regain your strength. We will send a couple of sea dragons to help you, and then we can hide you amongst them as we fly over, that will shock Norgra when you reappear in Decagon."

"Misty, why don't you head back to the camp? I will settle Pulsar by the beach and join you later. You can tell Skye and his mum and sister that Pulsar is alive, I will catch some Reedonk and make out that I have been hunting?" suggested Argon

Arriving back at camp Misty went straight back to the area the decagon and sea dragons were in. There were a lot more dragons there now. They looked quite happy to be on an adventure, especially a land one for a change. One of them drew nearer and introduced himself.

"Hello, I am Vortex, team leader for this lot. What can we do to help? I've got two watching the caves the Elders are in, so we will know if they stir."

"Hello Vortex, Skye could you join us please, let's walk out of sight for a few minutes. Over there will do," and Misty headed towards some tall rocks and walked round behind them.

"What's up?" asked Skye as he joined Misty and |vortex.

"Skye, I have something to tell you, but I don't want the elders to see you. Your father Pulsar is alive and on the beach near the pinnacle. Now please mind block before you tell the world."

Trying not to roar with joy, Skye hopped from foot to foot flapping his wings till he hovered. "How do you know this? Is he alright? Where was he?"

"Slow down young 'un," said Vortex, "it seems you have had great news, but let Misty get a word in and she will tell you." Laughing, he went on, "now I can see why you wanted him out of sight, he's as giddy as a shoal of neons, mind, I don't blame you. It is good news for you. In what way can I help you Misty?"

"Pulsar needs some help till he is stronger," Misty explained what had happened to him. "I know you want to see him Skye, but if

Vortex could send two of his dragons to teach Pulsar to swim and breathe underwater, and fish of course, he can regain his strength. In the meantime, Skye, do you think your mother and sister could keep it a secret, or would they be too happy and give it away. I was thinking that perhaps we could sneak them to stay on the beach, and tell folk they have got some illness, to explain why they don't come out of your cave, you know them best,m which is it?"

Skye stopped cavorting around and thought, "I think they should go to my father, it would be cruel for them not to know, and star certainly couldn't hide it for long. She would have to tell someone, so I suggest I take them tonight after dark. I can be back well before dawn. I won't tell Star till we are halfway there, then she can screech all she wants to."

"I think it might be wise to pack what you want to take with you to Decagon and stay at the beach till we leave, you as well Skye. I have Argon and Vortex here as protection, and you have earned a break. But remember, the atmorphics and other creatures are around, not forgetting the wolfcrabs, so don't drop your guard," said Misty, "we will get things moving here, any emergencies mind link."

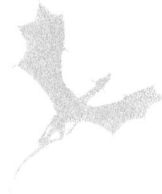

CHAPTER
14

Rainbow and Sabre were working on how to get the younglings free from the castle and to release Pearl. With all the sea dragons and his warriors, Rainbow had over six hundred dragons to fight Weld, plus the Guardians and the young dragons from the Cave of Destiny, but he had learned not to rely on sheer force, it would be subterfuge that would probably free them if possible, alongside the unexpected!

"I have summoned Blaze, Emerald, Aura and Topaz back with the other Cave of Destiny dragons. They should be here very soon, then we can really fine tune our plans, such as they are at the moment."

Ice was quietly sat in a corner making a drawing in the earth, and then she looked up and spoke. "I Know it   s not my place, but I've been thinking about the dungeons where the younglings are. I've made a map if it will help?"

Going to look, and just expecting to see a drawing, Sabre said "That is brilliant Ice!"

There was a full model made of frozen mud, showing the corridors and vaulted rooms that made up the dungeons. It even showed the secret tunnel to Natties garden, and the location of the stairways.

"Did you know there is a second tunnel behind this wall,?" said Ice.

"Under the curve of the stone steps into the dungeon was a wall, and behind it showed another large vaulted room with a tunnel leading into what looked like a really old part of the castle. I don't know where that goes, perhaps Beech and Elm know?"

"Rainbow, just look at this! If there is another way in, it changes everything doesn't it?"

When Rainbow had studied the map he agreed. "You are very brave and talented Ice, this is wonderful!"

Feeling rather proud, Ice said, "I wondered if we could sneak the younglings out of the castle into Natties garden and we put them on the nets and fly them over the wall quickly and silently, and that if we can find a way into the other room, we could hide Pearl there with Squib, so no-one could hurt her until she is rescued as well."

"Good thinking Ice, can you ask Beech, Elm and Squib if they can find a way into that room, and can Beech and Elm try and find out where that tunnel comes out, and is it big enough to hide adult dragons?" asked Rainbow.

"It's all questions of the unknown at the moment," said Sabre.

Just then Beech and Elm popped into everyone's view. "You wanted us?" asked Elm.

"We are here!" said Beech.

"Do you know the big room behind the curved staircase?" asked Rainbow.

Looking puzzled, the two popped out again, to reappear a few moments later.

"We had forgotten that place," said Beech, "it used to be a store room before Weld took the castle, bet no-one has told him!"

"Is there another way in?" asked Sabre.

"We can show you one way, but I can't remember how they got stuff into the store room. We will search for you. Who is coming to the way in from the inside then?" replied Elm.

"We will never fit," laughed Rainbow, "so it will have to be you Ice, I'm afraid".

"Can you message Squib where to meet you and please take care of them both," he asked the Tree Elves, "and yourselves of course."

"Ha ha" We're dead remember, no-one can hurt us," and leading Ice out of the garden they vanished into the dark.

"You know, it's the waiting that is the worst," said Rainbow, "not being able to plan in detail. I heard from Meteor, they have set out to return with the lost dragons, they can only be as quick as the slowest ones. He wanted to split into two groups and get the quickest and fittest back here to help. I told him to stay as close together as possible, with their numbers they are bound to attract some sort of predator, and the lost ones won't have any experience with them."

Rae, Topaz and Emerald look at Blaze. "They have found them. Yes, the eggs hatched safely with \pearls' help and they are now younglings, but Weld had a terrible plan for them, so we are going in!" said Blaze.

"Thank Draco for that," said Topaz, "we will be needed, and the young dragons?"

"They are wanted as well, we had better tell them," said Blaze, "this is not a game any more, and they are all about to become guardians and warriors before they are really ready. Emerald, can you get them all together please? I don't want to mind link as I am still getting news from Rainbow, oh and Misty and Meteor and a lot of other dragons are setting out from that land of Skyes. They will be part of something not seen for many years. A full dragon wing. Let's hops enough survive to tell their hatchlings."

When the young dragons had gathered, Blaze explained what was happening, and Weld's evil plan for the younglings.

"We have no choice but to go and get them, they are our own, our brothers and sisters, even if not, as dragons we protect our own. Do not be mistaken in thinking because you took out a swarm of goblins it will be easy! It's a risk you will take with your lives. Draco forbid we lose any of you, or you are maimed, or lose a wing, but it must be done or dragon kind is doomed. You have all been in the Cave of Destiny and know what is to come. Those with the gifts of healing and nurturing will hold positions away from the battle to come. To help those who need it. Those who are fastest will be delivering aid where needed, fire chillies, estra flame power, whatever has to be done and the rest of us will follow orders - to the letter - no heroics!"

There is a plan in place and we will obey it. Do you understand?!"

"Now go and think about your destinies, and if you need any advice, come and talk to us. Sometimes our path is not clear and guidance is needed. There is no fault in that; I'm just sorry you are being pushed into this position."

Leaving the young ones to their thoughts, Blaze, Emerald, Topaz and Rae went off to let them mull it over.

"We have quite a few who are good warrior material," said Rae, "Young Rock for one!"

"They will be fine, I know Rainbow will keep them as rearguard and messengers behind the senior warrior positions," Topaz said and went on, "let's get something to eat and see what other news is coming in. We will get them all fed and then clean up. We must leave no trace that we were here."

"If a goblin patrol were to come here and find traces, it could lead to the Destiny Cave being discovered."

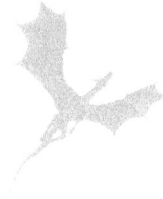

CHAPTER
15

While Skye and his family were re-uniting on the beach, back at the caves the dragons were sorting themselves into family groups. The elderley and the young were having it explained about the nets that had been brought.

"There is a sound reason for using these," said Misty, "you older ones will have the job of keeping the young ones in line and are not playing about. We can fly higher and faster if they keep reasonably still. That will leave the other dragons as out riders protecting and spelling the ones carrying the nets, Any questions?"

"I have one or two," came a voice from behind them. "Who is deciding on this, and who is in charge here? Asked Norgar nastily, "I thought I was the leader here!"

Vortex and Argon stepped between Norgra and Misty talons extended, in defence of their princess.

"As the senior ranked dragon here, I have asked your people who they wanted as temporary leader for the journey to Decagon, which they have all voted on. And, they have honoured me with their choice. So! Under dragon law, of which you have been conveniently and consistently breaking, you are no longer leader, and when we get back to Decagon, Rainbow and Pearl, Sabre and Coral are our dragon leaders, and all answer to them. So, you and your so-called Council must decide, are you coming or are you staying here? Decide! We will leave when the sun starts to sink below the horizon, then a lot of the trip will be done in the cool of the night, Oh, and before we go any further, you can only carry water with you and a small bag of personal items, not gold, gems or anything heavy" Do you understand?"

And leaving them with jaws open. Misty walked away.

"Well that told him," chuckled Argon, "What's the betting he will try and take his treasure with him."

"It's inevitable," laughed Vortex, "I think we should let him try and then make him, and no doubt the others, drop it all into the sea, that will stop him from noticing Pulsar amongst us."

"We should reach the first island by moonrise," said Misty, "we will give them a rest and then head for island two, and everyone can sleep there and feed up on fish before we set off.. We should be back at Decagon by evening of the second day all being well! Any trouble from Norgar we leave him here or maroon him on Gushyberry Island. Oh, and Argon, I need you to teach all the new dragons to watch out for atmorphics and wolf crabs and how to help you."

It was as the sun started to sink, about two hundred dragons gathered together, in a quiet mood by the adults and suppressed excitement by the younglings. There were ten nets all laid on the ground waiting for their precious cargo. One of the mothers looked nervous as she asked, "Are these safe and how strong are they?"

"The merfolk who make them, use them to catch fish bigger than us," answered Vortex, "and we use them quite often to carry younglings about quickly. They are safe enough, feel this one here, how strong it is. You can help carry one if you want."

Reassured, the mother went over to the others and told them what had been said.

"Time to load, come on young 'uns. I want six of you on each net and three adults. Sort yourselves into net groups and step onto the nets, now sit down comfortably and no messing around", instructed

Vortex. "Right I need the adults to go round the first net, see those straps there, they will fit over your wings onto your backs, like this. Now the weight is spread and they don't interfere with your flying. If you feel you are getting tired, call one of us to take over and give you a break. Don't be proud you are all doing your bit."

"Norgra, what are you doing?", asked Meteor as he saw him go and sit on a net. "You are fit enough to fly. We are not ferrying you around. Go over there and put a net strap on, you can do the first leg of the trip carrying!"

"But I'm...", and before he could go further, Argon opened his wings and bared his teeth, "You are a dragon the same as the rest of us, and you and your cronies can do the same,now get on with it!"

At last when everyone was in place and on the command "Lift", all the nets slowly rose into the air and the dragons were on the move to a new life in a rich and fertile land.

The warriors had been flying as outsiders checking that everything was going well, and as they approached, the sight of the sea had all the land dragons spellbound. At this stage Argon signalled the warriors, who flew off in twos and fours scouting round, and as they set off over the water all the different groups rejoined the exodus. This way, no-one noticed the extra dragons amongst them. Skye went scouting ahead with Meteor , and Pulsar, Cloud and Star mixed in with the sea dragons at the rear.

To the younglings, it was an adventure of a lifetime, and the oldest and youngest were able to look about at leisure because they were being net carried.

"Why is the water moving?" asked one of the younglings.

One of the sea dragons answered, "It is the moon, she moves the water in one direction, and then another. We can use the directions to make moving around easier, from one land to another and it keeps the air in the water to keep it fresh."

"Oh, I think I would like to be a sea dragon."

"You will have your chance to decide when you have been to the Cave of Destiny youngling, and then it will be clear to you."

So the journey went on, with warriors taking their turns at carrying the nets.

"Why are you all flying round, and keeping a lookout?" asked an elder, "what is there out here that is so dangerous?"

"Atmorphics, they are land, sea and air creatures, and as deadly as they come," said Argon, "they appear to be beautiful till they get in range. It is a terrible thing to see, they suck your innards out and tear you to pieces while you are still alive, the last thing left is the scream, so keep your eyes open and wits about you, they can come out of the sea or air very easily."

"Poppycock", muttered Norgra, it's just a tale to scare you all. I for one don't believe it. I'm getting tired, will someone take over - please!"

"Can you hang on for a short while, we are almost at the first island rest stop, then we will all eat and drink. Some of the warriors will keep air patrols watching out though." answered Argon.

Soon in the distance an island came into view. It was lush and green and had gushyberry trees all over it.

Argon said The fruits on the trees will provide food and drink for you all. Can you elders make sure the younglings all eat something, but don't overdo it, too many first time can give you bellyache."

And, leading the exodus of dragons Argon headed for a large glade amongst the trees and landed.

Once the nets had been lowered to the ground the younglings all wanted to explore. So, while adults picked fruit for them, they charged around like spring rabbits.

Soon hunger took over and everyone was settled and eating, all except the air patrol

"These are wonderful!" Some of the dragons who had never seen gushyberries before marvelled at the fruits.

"Is this what is waiting for us? Is Decagon all green? Is there plenty of water? Some of the younglings have never seen a river, are there many there?

Many of the younglings and the older dragons had so many questions. During the flight they had had time to think and wonder about this new land they were going to.

After about an hour, they all prepared to leave, with different adults doing the net carrying. They all left the island and headed off again. It was about three hours to the next island but only the Decagon dragons knew that. Since they didn't trust Norgra and his cronies, the less they knew the better. They were making good time as the winds were blowing their way and they didn't have to stop and make the islands this time. Argon joined Misty and pointed out a distant speck in the sky.

"I've told Meteor and Skye to warn the others, but there is only one other thing I know of that can fly this far out to sea, an atmorphic. We need to reach the next island as quickly as possible. I've told the spare warriors to help with the nets so we can go faster. Is it much further?"

"It is about as far as the atmorphic is, but in the other direction, so we are headed away from the creature. Let's hope we can land in time," said Misty, and calling to all the dragons, she urged them to fly faster. As they all understood there was danger threatening, there was a sense of urgency about them. It was a race against time.

Slowly, but surely, the distant spec grew larger, but they could see that the island was appearing on the opposite horizon.

Misty called out, "There is a large meadow in the centre of the island. As soon as we land, I want you all to take cover in the treeline. Warriors I need you to protect the perimeter, don't show yourselves. Is there anyone without fire chillies? I have some spare ones, come and get them on landing," And so the race began

Would they land in time?

It was a bit of a bumpy landing for those in the nets, but they scrambled free and hid in the trees. Most bunched together for mutual protection, but Norgra and his cronies headed away from the rest.

"This could be our chance," he told them, "If we take control of that creature, we have the ultimate power. We can mind link and take it over, then use it to control the others. I want that jewel of Princess Mistys', and we can take over Decagon with our mind powers and that "Thing" it will be easy!"

So, waiting and watching they plotted.

"Do we let them know that we know what they are up to," said Meteor.

"No," said Misty, wearily, "let them be the engineers of their own fate, and a lesson to any others who think to betray us." And turning to the other dragons told them, "The younglings don't need to see this, there is a pool of water near here, I will take them there to play, but I will return immediately to join you."

So, taking the younglings to the pool a very sad and tired dragon Princess left them there, playing, with instructions to stay there until the adults brought food. She then returned to her Decagon dragon friends to face what was to come

It wasn't long before a great shadow fell over the meadow as the atmorphic arrived overhead. It was a fascinating creature, almost hypnotic, with the flickering coloured lights running up and down its tentacles and body. It had a smile on its fish looking face and looked beautiful. Stepping out of the treeline Norgra and his men linked minds and projected the thoughts of control to the.atmorphic, which came slowly closer to them. Very gently it placed a tentacle on each dragon's neck, and then, without warning, barbs appeared on the tentacles and punctured the veins in their necks and the lights flickered faster. Then the smile turned into a great gaping maw, tearing them apart as it was sucking them dry. It was a horrific sight.

There was a collective gasp from the other dragons. It was enough to turn the atmorphics' attention towards them, but Misty and the Decagon warriors were ready.

Stepping out they unleashed a terrible wall of flame. Imagine the power of eighteen adult dragons. They incinerated the beast in seconds. Turning away Misty saw Pulsar there with the warriors.

"You didn't need to join in."

"Yes I did," he said, "they were my dragons and as despicable as they were, they have been avenged and I have helped to protect my innocent dragons, perhaps the flames will cleanse their memories of that sight, thank you."

"Perhaps," said Vortex who was with them, "Pulsat might want to cheer his dragons up by letting them see he is alive. There is only a scorch mark left on the grass. If we light a fire before the younglings come back, that will be enough to make us all feel good, and, if we catch some nice big fish for dinner?"

And so, it was, the night became a celebration of Pulsars' return with lovely baked fish for supper, and a good night's sleep.

The next morning saw a very happy group of dragons. Their beloved leader was back. All the families were together and they had a new beginning of freedom to look forward to.

"I think we can spend a while and teach them all to swim and fish. It will be safer when we are over the water and if any atmorphics come we can tip them into the water while we fight them," suggested Vortex to Argon.

Agreeing, the time taken would be with it, they mind linked with all the dragons and explained what they were doing.

"We will put you into groups with Argon, Vortex, Pulsar, Meteor and Skye, and any who are a bit scared Star can help with them. They should also be taught how to block the goblin smell as well, just in case!" said Misty.

After a good feed of fish and a reminder not to look at the lights of an atmorphic if one came in range, the whole exodus set off again.

"It is only a short trip to the Sea Dragon island as the wind is still with us. Now everyone is free of the threat of Norgra and his cohorts and Pulsar is back amongst us, this will be a happy journey," said Argon.

It was a happy bunch of dragons that set off for Sea Dragon Island and it was if the fates were helping them. The wind picked up and helped blow them straight and true to the next island for a short rest and to let the younglings play in the water for a while, practising their new found skills.

Approaching the land after an uneventful leg of the journey, Misty contacted Rainbow. *"We are almost back, where do you want us to take everyone, they are all safe now we have got rid of the corrupted ones."*

"Home Valley," replied Rainbow, *"you can meet up with Aura, Hope and Peri there. Ask Pulsar and his mate Comet to help look after them, there will be enough guardians to help show what is dangerous, and explain to them all what's happening, younglings included. They all need to know what is going on, as well as being on the lookout for goblins and grawks. Can you join us here in Volcano Valley, when you have rested of course?"*

"Blaze, did you get all that? I want you all to come to Volcano valley as soon as possible please. We will all meet up there and plan."

"No problems," was the answer from Blaze, *"it's been very quiet since the goblins. We are on our way now, we will see you soon."*

"Aura, can you hand the protection of the younglings over to Comet and Pulsars' dragons, and you, Hope and Peri join us when they are sorted."

And, in an open message he told them all, *"We are going to rescue everyone, and I am asking for volunteers. Those who cannot fight, or are guardians or younglings must stay behind and protect the future of Dragonkind on Decagon. That duty is sacred. You have all been told what your destiny is, except the new dragon family joining us. They need to rest and learn, and guard the younglings for the future. May Draco protect us in the time to come, and may the dragon parents finally meet their young!"*

As Pulsars' family approached the land, they were all curious to see their new homes. There were "Oohs" and "Aahs" from the younglings and pleased smiles from the adults.

"Not much further now," said Argon.

And, as they flew across the grassy plains a voice called, "Can we all fly in and not be carried any further!"

"Of course," said Misty, "I should have thought of that."

So, they landed and everyone had a chance to stretch their legs. The younglings were all rolling around in the grass, all giddy and excited, they had never seen anything like it.

"Wait till they see snow," said Misty to Pulsars' mate, Comet.

"Snow?" she queried, "Even I haven't seen that!"

"Well you will find out for sure, when you start exploring. Right, are we ready? Let's go to see your new home."

And like a swarm of bees, the multi-coloured and multi-sized flight of dragons took off over the rolling hills and forests till they came eventually to Home Valley, and with a slow curve of flight they came to rest.

There were many dragons waiting to welcome them. The younglings all ran to greet the newcomers, who were just a bit overwhelmed.

It was over. They were free.

In a beautiful land, and made welcome as a family. Many of the mothers had a tear in her eye, while watching the younglings intermingle with their new friends.

"You must be hungry," said a lovely gold dragon. "I am Aura, this is Peri and this is Hope, we are warriors here to help the guardians look after everyone, and you must be Pulsar and Comet. Welcome brothers and sisters, come and see your new home, gushyberries younglings?"

That brought forth a great cheer from them, and dashing to where the fruits were piled up, they happily got down to eating the gushyberries.

"We have a meal ready for you, or do you want to catch your own?"

"Whatever you have done will be wonderful," said Comet, "we are truly grateful, you've saved Skye and Pulsar, got rid of Norgra and given us a new start in a beautiful place in the home of our ancestors. Draco did hear our plea for help."

And chatting happily they went to join the others and rebuild the bond of Dragonkind.

Aura explained to Comey and Pulsar that the warriors, when they had rested a bit and eaten, would be joining up with Rainbow in Volcano Valley, but they would have the guardians and a few others to teach what was needed. The younglings will quickly learn from ours, but you and Comet will take over here for Rainbow;"

"We ask that you protect our future and yours, while we fight for the stolen ones, and return them to their families!"

It seemed no time at all before all the warriors gathered ready to set off. The guardians were ready to help with the transition, and then they were off to Volcano Valley to rendezvous with Rainbow.

Travelling at a fair speed, the warriors and the young dragons from the Cave of Destiny, flying high and keeping a wary eye out for grawks. They made good time and soon could see faint traces of smoke in the distance.

Then, Topaz spotted a shape below them and mind linking, *"There's a pair of grawks down there, they have been shadowing us for a while. Blaze if you head to Rainbow, Rae, Emerald and I will take them out, then they cannot give us away. You're the strongest Blaze, and Rainbow needs you. Wait till we pass that outcrop over there and we will break away and ambush them from there."*

Reluctantly Blaze agreed. *"I never have any fun! See you at the valley."*

Waiting behind the outcrop it wasn't long before they heard the flapping of large wings. Much faster than a dragon's strong leisurely beat. Emerald started flying as though she was trying to catch up with a group in the distance. Spotting her, the grawks were trying to catch up and get either side of her, that's when Rae and Topaz struck.

They came up behind the grawks and mentally told Emerald they were in place, she veered off and circled round, and then they struck. A jet of flame hit each one of the grawks and cooked them! Emerald's quick thinking caught them as they were dropping.

"No point in leaving any traces, we can either eat 'em or put them on the perimeter of the volcano as victims. He he he."

"We will see what Shadow suggests, it is his job to scare goblins and things off." suggested Topaz

Approaching the valley from the seaward side so no-one could see them, Blaze and the young warrior from the cave came into land. Some of the young adults were puzzled.

"What are those things on the rocks and swimming around, they were quite strange?" asked Rock.

"Those are mer-people and they make the nets we use. We barter gushyberries for them, and their shape is very handy. They have hands that can make many things and some can change their fish tails for funny shaped legs, so they can walk out of the water like us. They may be puny but they are very clever and have some deadly weapons to fight with."

"What sort of weapons?"

"Long straight branches sharpened like claws. Tridents they call them, and ones with sharp shells as cutting or stabbing weapons called spears. You will be very respectful to these people. They protect our seaward side and we protect them from the landward. Always look after your allies."

"Someone's coming," called one of the younger ones.

They all turned to watch, and three more shapes came into land.

"Who is that?" asked Rock.

"It's Rae, Emerald and Topaz, they sorted out the grawks that were following us," said Blaze, "that none of you saw, and I've told you that your lives depend on you being alert and aware. Anything moving or out of place, tell us!"

By the time the three dragons had landed Rainbow and Shadow had joined them.

"Well now, look at that, cooked grawk! Haven't had one of them in years, they give us a wide berth here." Shadow said.

"Perhaps you would like them," said Topaz, "we brought them along so there was no trace of us passing. We thought you would know the best use for them."

"Oh, I know exactly what to do with them," said Shadow, smiling, taking the roasted birds he headed towards his cave, chuckling.

Rainbow looked over all the dragons there, "Thank you, and here come Aura, Perri and Hope with news of our newest family members. If any of you have any wounds or hurts, Peri is a healer and can help you."

One surprise awaited Rainbow. Thirty dragons arrived with Aura.

"Rainbow, this is Pulsar and some of his dragons, they insist on fighting for their new family."

Stepping forward with the other dragons, Pulsar bowed to Rainbow saying, "You are my leader and this is my family now. Don't deny us the chance to honour your kindness, and be as one."

"Brothers, you are more than welcome to help, but don't put yourselves at risk," said Rainbow. "Blaze, I'm putting Pulsar with you, look after him."

And he put each of Pulsars' dragons with an experienced warrior. "It's not because we don't trust you as fighters, but because you don't even know yet what a goblin or a grawk looks like, let alone an ogre!"

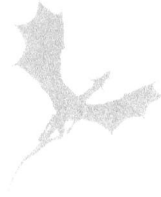

CHAPTER
16

S tanding in Volcano Valley, Rainbow looked out at about six hundred dragons, he linked with Pearl and showed her the fantastic sight.

"These are our family, and we are coming to get you tonight! Warn only Ice, Squib, Elm and Beech, then the younglings won't give anything away with excitement or fear, but they must be silent and obey any orders once we start. Can you send Elm and Beech to me please?"

To the astonishment of a lot of dragons, Elm and Beech popped into view. Mind you, they were just as shocked to see so many dragons.

"Good grief," said Elm, "That's a lot of dragonzez!"

"What can we do?" asked Beech.

Rainbow spread his wings and called, "Dragons" and instantly everyone was watching and listening."These are Elm and Beech; they are our own heroes and are helping us. So don't mistake them for anything but friends. Now that you have seen them, all eat and rest; we will tell you the plan in a short while. Please keep noise and movement to a minimum so no-one gets hurt in the dark, when it comes."

Taking Elm and Beech to meet his warrior leaders, Rainbow asked "Did you find the door to the big room?"

"We done better than that," said \beech, "we've found a big tunnel as well! It's in the old part. I reckon you dragons had the castle first from the size of it, and it comes out of the opposite wall in the west courtyard. The door to one of the rooms is in one of the cells opposite your Pearl! I think they were store rooms originally and Weld had them changed over. Good job he didn't know about the tunnels. This should make capturing the castle easy. Sneak the young 'uns and your lady Pearl out, get them away to safety, and put some of your lot inside, through the tunnels, you can get them inside and out! Like smoking goblins out of a kitchen! Do you want us to find out how many goblins there are and where they are? And see if his nibs has got any booby traps set up. . We can set them off; it's not as though they can kill us, is it? We drive him crazy like that, so he won't be expecting anyone but us. I'm so looking forward to seeing his face when he realises his prisoners have gone, and it's just adult dragons he is facing!"

So, giggling to themselves the two selfless ghosts popped out of sight to do a goblin count.

As the evening drew near, the warrior dragon leaders were planning with Rainbow and Sabre. Misty and Peri were making suggestions. Topaz and some of the others were checking on medical supplies. No-one was kidding themselves that they would escape without any injuries. Fire chillies were being ferried from the growing area, and great mounds were ready to be used. An average dragon could eat about two hundred fire chillies when readying for battle, and store as many again in their pouches, that would give them at least two hours of flames, and with huge supplies on hand with the young warriors to re-supply them, they could fire and claw for days.

It was an unusually quiet gathering that evening, as everyone awaited orders. Skye and his dad were with the warrior dragons, quietly talking about what had happened to the Decagon dragons and their families as well, each one worried about the safety of the other.

Now Weld was in his castle reading an ancient grimoire, when a disturbance drew his attention. "What's all the noise about!" he demanded. "You know it must be peaceful when I am reading."

A goblin came rushing in. "We are so sorry, o great one, but these ghosts are at it again. They've locked the armoury door from the inside, and we can't get in! And, they've opened all the taps on the oil that was for boiling and pouring over the walls. It has all run down the steps of the turrets and we can't get up them!"

"Those obnoxious ghosts have driven me mad. They have no respect for me! They should be on their knees with gratitude at being around my presence. I will make them beg for mercy when I kill them for a second time. You tell the captain of the guard to make sure all the shredding blades are still in their places for firing, and put a guard on them!"

Now, listening inside the walls to this, Beech and Elm were gleeful. They didn't know about any shredding blades or where they were, and now Weld was getting his goblins to show them where they were. All round the castle walls were these odd big boxes and the goblin and the captain of the guard went and checked them all.

Beech was invisible and stuck his head through the lid of the box to see what was in them. He soon came back out.

"We have to warn Rainbow," he whispered to Elm.

Popping up in front of Rainbow, they told him what they had done so far.

"But that's not all" was Beech's warning, "all around the walls are boxes. In them is a machine with springs and it's full of star shaped blades that are so sharp they will maim." And pulling at a shiny bit of metal he pulled out a star.

"As far as I can see, when the springs fire these off they start spinning and can cause a lot of damage, especially to wings! How can we get rid of them?"

"I've got an idea," said Topaz, "but I need to talk to Blaze. I will be back to you."

126

Going over to where Blaze was checking her lists, Topaz asked her, "You know when we found out Squib was able to become invisible, I was wondering how many of the others have the talent, but kept quiet about it, so they could have some fun?"

"There's a thought," said Blaze, "I bet there are a few. That could come in very handy don't you think?"

"I asked because I have an idea about these star boxes. Do you remember when we were younglings and we sneaked into the leader's cave and pinched them chickens he had flamed?"

"Ooh yes," said Blaze, "and then we covered the wooden chest up with snakeshead lily sap. It glued the chest up solid and he couldn't open it at all."

"Well if we had some small invisible dragons with a big supply of snakeshead lily sap, they could just glue the boxes shut. It's clear and it sets instantly. So, they won't know till they want to use them."

Topaz smiled at the thought of her suggestion and said, "Blaze. Ice could freeze a few perhaps?"

"I didn't know she could vanish as well," said Rainbow.

"Oh yes, we found out a while ago which leads me to believe that she and Squib are brother and sister. Another thing, have you noticed he is slowly getting darker? I think he is going to end up black. You know what that means, don't you?" said Topaz. "He and Ice are your two younglings. Ice is slowly getting the silver/mother of pearl sheen that Pearl has and you and Sabre are both black dragons that reflect the light and become rainbows. Wait till pearl finds out, she will be delighted!"

Topaz joined the others. "Well I have found nine invisibles. I've asked Coral to check on her younglings. They didn't want to admit it till I said there was a dangerous top-secret mission on the go, and then they were all popping in and out of sight to prove they could do it. Draco blesses them!"

"Right Blaze, please take charge of them and show them some control techniques and also how to safely use snakeshead lily sap without glueing their wings together," asked Rainbow. "Also, I need you to arrange that the other younglings are kept occupied and out of mischief. I thought we could get them to bring fire chillies to different spots as resupply points."

And with this Rainbow detailed everyone with their missions.

"Peri you are in charge of the scouts and any injuries. The scouts will be doing patrols from now on to keep an eye on the castles' occupants. Keep the reports coming into Sabre please!"

"Emerald I need you to lead a group into the large tunnel; you will have Elm, Beech and Rae with you as well as another group of warriors. There will be about eighty of you all told. I've picked you because Pearl knows you all and I need her to give your mental pictures to the younglings, who have no idea of what is happening yet. So, familiar faces will help keep them calm to get them out as quickly and quietly as you can, then defend the tunnel."

"I need you Blaze, to lead the invisibles to the castle and use the hidden entrance to get them into the castle. There they can vanish and go seal up those star boxes so they can't be used against us. We don't need any wings damaging tonight. Keep them safe Blaze."

"Argon, Vortex and Misty, I want you to take a flight to the north side and wait there."

"Hope, Pulsar and Skye, I want you to take a flight to the west side and wait. Hope, I want you to make sure Ice and Squid And Nattie get out safely."

"Sabre, Aura and Meteor will take a flight to the south side and I will take Topaz and Rock to the east side with a flight."

"Everyone, there will be ogres, grawks, goblins and who knows what in there, so all be careful. There are one hundred and eighty five dragons on sky duty, if anyone is injured, drop out and go to Shadow if you can. If not, some of the sky patrol will help you, and refill your positions."

"Everything is on hold till the younglings and pearl and the invisibles are out of the castle completely, then we block the exits and the group with Emerald will slowly work upwards clearing everything in their path."

"Watch out for each other, and beware of booby traps, When they start moving upwards, we will attack! It is claws and jaws everyone, seek and destroy. Make it quick and clean, but keep your wits about you."

"Blaze, with your team of invisibles go now and start your mission, don't let anyone get careless, your lives depend on looking out for each other. Everyone else to your positions and wait for my call.."

"Rae and Emerald get ready to enter the tunnel on my say so. Silence is imperative if we don't want to cause panic."

Pearl, can you give the younglings some warning and tell them to be as quiet as a hunting dragon. Not long now till you are all free. Patience, just a bit longer. Have you got Squib and Ice with you, and nattie! Keep them close to you.

Blaze and her team were quite enjoying themselves sneaking up on the guarded boxes, and plastering them with the snakehead lily sap. They nearly came to grief when one guard sat on a box and was stuck to it. Rather than have him shout for help and give them away, Blaze gave him a quick bite on the back of his neck and silenced him for good. Since he was stuck to the box it just looked as though he was asleep, but the younglings stuffed their tails in their mouths to stop them from laughing out loud.They soon realised it was not a game but deadly serious and carried out their mission in absolute silence. It took a good while to check everywhere for the boxes for they dare not miss any. At last Blaze was satisfied they were all safe.

"OK team we are out of here, Go quietly back to the tunnel and stay invisible till we are out of the castle."

In silent procession they retraced their steps when they heard voices.

"Get into the alcoves," thought Blaze to them,and taking the smallest ones under her wings, she held them safe. In a moment two goblins came down some stairs chuntering to themselves.

"Why should we have to make sure them dragons is clean, going in the big pots will sort that out. It's not as though he will taste them anyway. Just imagine dragon stew with thick gravy, fair makes your mouth water, doesn't it?", and heading down the corridor they turned a corner and went out of sight and hearing.

"Right that does it!" thought Blaze and messaging to Emerald she told her and the others to come fast and silent. Turning to her team she told them to go back down the tunnel, stand to one side and let the warriors see you as they go past. Hurry and get out of here. Go straight to Hope. Tell her it is time to be ready and then go back to Volcano Valley, and, I mean all of you. No hanging around, if you do you will put us all at risk. Go on now, hurry, but quietly, and leaving no trace all the dragons left.

Blaze told Rainbow what had been heard. *I'm following, there's only two so I can deal with them and give us some time."*

"Take care Blaze," thought Rainbow, *"Draco be with you."*

Going down the corridor, Blaze followed the goblins. With the smell they made it easy to do, when she came to a junction she stopped and listened and could quite clearly hear a voice of authority say "I don't care what you have been told, it's too cold for them to swim, ridiculous idea and most are asleep anyway, go away!"

"Now seez 'ere your majesty in chains, I don't fink it it's any fink to do with you anymore, so just tell them young 'uns to behave and do what we tell 'em before we open the door."

Blaze couldn't resist it, "Is your majesty having problems? Can I help in any way?"

Opening the door which the goblins though locked Blaze slowly materialized and appeared in all her scarlet glory, advancing on the two goblins who were struck dumb with fear.

She spoke again, "Pearl my dear sister, it's time."

"Now you were saying you horrible little creatures," and with one blow of her wing she hit them into the wall with all the pent-up anger she had held back, so hard that they left a big 'Splat' green mark on the wall as they slid down.

"That feel better?" asked Pearl, "How long have we got?"

"Minutes I think," said Blaze, "come on let's get the young 'uns out of here."

They undid the bolt on the door and opened it. All the younglings gathered round for instructions.

"This is Blaze, she is to be obeyed instantly, if she tells you anything. Right out of here, which way Blaze?"

Then around the corner ran Emerald and the warriors

"Pearl, thank goodness.there's no time to waste, there are twenty warriors to escort you out of here. We will hold the fort (ha ha) till you are clear and free."

Splitting into two groups, Pearl, Blaze and the younglings set off down the corridor to the tunnel entrance, while the warriors checked out the area including the steps up to the next floor. Hurrying as quickly as they could, the younglings were soon at the tunnel entrance. Wait was the command, let us check it out first.

Having checked with Hope and the others that there was no-one on the battlements, and it was clear to run to the trees, the warrior leader told them, *"When you leave the entrance, go right, stay as close to the wall as you can and don't make a sound. Get to the trees and sit down till everyone is out. Do you all understand? Mind link only"*

So it was, the younglings hugged the wall and got into the cover of the trees. The excitement was incredible; they were out of the castle for the first time in their lives,

Hope did a head count; there were twenty six younglings plus nattie, Squib and Ice. Linking with Rainbow, she told him they are all here.

"Right" he replied and decided to get them out of there as quickly as possible, so he asked Peri to send some of the sky patrol to carry them to volcano valley, out of the range of Weld.

"Wait till the next cloud bank comes over and grab them out of here before the new moon rises, which by looking at those clouds won't be long at all. I will see if I can increase the clouds and speed them up a bit. Get ready to move quickly!" And, concentrating hard he slowly increased the speed and size of the dark cloud bank.

"Go now younglings, Not a sound. You are going to be picked up by the warriors and taken to Volcano Valley, just co-operate and be as quiet as you can."

With the sound of flapping wings about fifty warriors flew down, gently grasped a youngling each and took off again, heading for Volcano Valley, the extra warriors were escorting them all.

Pearl and Hope embraced.

"I am so glad that you are free again, Rainbow is by the east wall if you want to go to him. Go before the action starts. The warriors here can guard the tunnel for escapees. Go on, go to him."

Flexing her wings, Pearl took off, taking care to fly round the castle and not across it so that she wouldn't be seen. She finally met up with Rainbow again, and Rock and Topaz went out of the way to let them re-unite in private.

Meanwhile having cleared the steps to the next level, Emerald, Rae and the warriors met no opposition.

"That's funny, I would have expected the alarm to be raised by now," said Rae.

It wasn't till they reached the kitchen level that they understood. There were Beech, Elm and Blaze.

"Hello, what kept you?" said Elm, "we have been having fun."

"It seems," said Blaze, "our two heroes here have been putting things in the goblins' dinner and they are all fast asleep, so we have a clear run to the next floor. Beech and Elm are going to scout ahead, off you pop lads.", and off they vanished to reappear almost instantly.

"There are goblins coming down the stairs and have two grawks with them. But, they have an ogre with them as well!"

"Oh joy," said Blaze, "let's make them welcome."

Moving across to a large kitchen trolley, Blaze very elegantly laid upon it and crossed her front claws, closed her eyes and waited.

The others all took cover and waited to see the legendary Blaze in action. Coming into the kitchen, the five goblins, the ogre and the grawks stopped dead.

"Strewth, he's cooked one already. It looks almost alive don't it. Said the ogre walking over to the trolley, the others followed, Just as the ogre was about to poke the 'cooked dragon' it opened its eyes and asked "Wasn't I in the oven long enough."

Well that of course panicked the goblins and grawks, but ogres are made of sterner stuff, and although he flinched, he was more curious than scared, I mean, who is frightened by their dinner?

"I take it you take a lot longer to brown and crisp up then?" said the ogre.

"Oh yes," said Blaze, "feel, I'm still all soft and juicy!"

Stepping forward, he poked Blaze, who immediately grasped his hand, pulled him close and turned into an incandescent ball of flame.

"Oh dear, I think he's a tad overcooked now," said Blaze as she switched off her flames,,

Seeing the ogre crisped in seconds, the goblins and grawks made a dash for the door, but to no avail, the crossfire between two lots of dragons had them well cooked as well.

"If you can't stand the heat, stay out of the kitchen lads, heh heh," chuckled Blaze. "Elm, Beech, can you see what the noise is about please?" And, poof! They were gone.

Back in seconds, they reported that the alarm was raised, the drugged goblins had been missed, as well as the well cooked patrol. A search was made for them and Weld could be ranting and raving in the upper floors.

"Let's go and see how far we get before they realise we are here, and the younglings are gone, heh heh," chuckled Elm.

When Rainbow checked on their whereabouts, he made his decision.

"Ok. This is it my friends, May Draco be with you, and we will all dragon roar at the end, but for now, let us tell Weld we are here. Let's have the biggest roar in history, NOW!"

And the mightiest sound you will ever have heard burst forth from over six hundred dragons.

"What on earth is that!" snarled Weld, "it is from outside."

Stomping to the window arch he saw an incredible sight. Dragons everywhere! Rushing onto the tower parapet he looked and on all four sides the castle was surrounded by dragons, with even more circling the skies above and another group coming from the volcanos.

"Where have they all come from, I've never seen so many dragons. Well if they have come for their hatched eggs they will be upset. I have a good mind to eat some in front of them. Guards! Go get me two of them little dragons. I'll threaten to kill them all if they don't back off! Guards' you cowardly goblins, hiding no doubt, I will rip your heads off when this is over, And where are my ogres. Is no-one answering me?" raged Weld.

Going to the circular staircase he looked down to see an army of dragons inexorably climbing the steps.

"What! How have they got in?Treachery! I'll kill you all for this, how dare you disrespect me! You bunch of old dragons, you should be obeying my every wish, it's not as though you have minds of your own!" raved Weld

Heading for the higher staircase, he climbed to the next level, barring the doors behind him, quite forgetting Elm and Beech didn't need doors. So, they danced along behind him laughing at his misery.

Reaching the next tower level Weld checked outside at what was happening, and as he showed his face a dragon nearby let off a huge blast of fire at him. Quickly ducking out of sight he went to the next level, this was no better, as he could see all the dragons around him. Cursing them all he looked for a way out and wasn't helped when Elm and Beech popped into sight laughing at him.

"You miserable ghosts think you will have the last laugh, well you won't, those kid dragons and that hoity toity Pearl will die before they can be rescued." snarled Weld.

"Is that so?" said Elm, "and with you up here and them down there how do you figure that out? Pardon me asking your honour the question, me being stupid and all,"

His mind on other things Weld answered Elm without thinking.

"All the dungeons downstairs are soaked in fire oil so if those dragons come near there, they will be the ones to kill their own offspring, as one good fire blast will set it all on fire. Pity I didn't get a couple of them before this started."

Now while he had been countering, Beech had popped off to tell the dragons about the fire oil. Popping back into the tower he was in time to hear Weld say, "And not all secret passages are in the dungeons and inside walls."

Opening a door that led to the top level of the tower, inside, by the steps was a huge lever, using his great strength he pulled the lever and part of the staircase moved leading to another room and in it was a pair of very large grawks.

"Thought they had me trapped did they. We will see!"

Opening the window Weld put his hands into the leather straps round the grawks ankles and with no further ado they launched from the window taking Weld with them.

Suspended between the grawks, whose very powerful wings started to gain height, Weld began heading south.

Aura spotted him first and launched to attack with flames. Roaring with fury she engulfed the grawks and Weld in flames.

"Back, back." screamed Weld, and his two grawks loyal to the end dropped him on top of the tower before crashing to their deaths with feathers aflame.

Beating the flames out of his clothes, Weld was livid, but Aura wasn't done with him yet. Circling round the tower, she spouted flames whenever she saw him.

"You stole out eggs and you were going to eat them for their magic, you great lump of goblin dung! You are not fit to leave footprints on the earth!"

By the light of the new moon everything was lit up like daylight. But even though he was surrounded he was still spiteful enough to shout,"I've killed all your runts and Pearl as well; you will never get them back!"

Climbing back into a room he went into the corner and uncovered a wood box. It was a shredder box. Elm and Beech who had been safely watching from inside of the room immediately popped off and went to Sabre, he being the nearest dragon and told him about the box.

He sent an immediate mind link to all the dragons to pull back and flew up to get Aura who was so angry she hadn't listened.

Flying into her line of vision he forced her to pay attention, and they flew back to the south side of the castle.

"I'm so sorry Sabre, I wanted to destroy him!"

"Time enough for that, but we must keep everyone safe."

With the light of the moon and the flames from the castle, it was like daylight, so no-one noticed flickering lights in the distance.

Slowly they drew nearer.

"Looks like all the noise and light has attracted some attention," Rainbow warned everyone, "all of you stay in groups or get under cover, no noise. Eat some fire chillies while you can. They are atmorphics; all the new dragons stay close to the older ones, who will stop you making mistakes. These are lethal!"

Attracted by all the light they had been drawn inland to where the action was,in search of prey. The castle being lit up was an obvious target. As they circled the castle the only living thing was Weld.. Seeing them he was dumbfounded; he had never seen anything like them before. Curious, he looked out of the window, mesmerised by the lights he wanted to catch one, so he opened the lid of the box he was holding. Too late did he realise that he might have made a mistake as all the shredding stars launched from the box, firing into the atmorphic, spinning and shredding as they went.

The most unholy screech came from it as it was mortally wounded; even so it tried to attack back, shooting its barbed tentacles into the window, trying to get him, But its strength was fading fast and as life ebbed out of it, it plummeted to the ground. Not a pretty sight, from that height it splattered everywhere.

"No-one goes near it, they are toxic to the touch." warned Rainbow.

Weld, seeing a chance, climbed up onto the roof to get to the other side of the tower where there was a door and a staircase down, as Beech had locked the door on the outside of the room he had been in. It was his only way out. Running across the roof keeping his eye out for the dragons, he missed the large shape in the darkness of the clouds which were forming over the sky.

With his hand on the door knob Weld pulled at the door, but it was locked. Elm had thought of it and locked that one while Beech had done the other. Roaring with rage Weld pulled and tugged at the door to no avail, and as he realised he was trapped the dark shape began to flicker its lights, slowly increasing the speed.

They were really quite pretty, flickering along its tentacles, and then it struck! Hooking its barbed tentacles into Weld's flesh it started to drain him, sucking his blood with every pulse of light, and then another figure joined it. Much smaller but definitely an atmorphic, and then another. Two young ones were joining the feast, and slowly they tore Weld apart and ate him.

"Ugh", said Sabre, "a whole family of them, We can't let them escape, they will forever be hunting over the land if they realise there is a plentiful food source here."

"Dragons" said Rainbow, "ready your fire and slowly rise up, all together."

When all the dragons had formed an invincible circle round the atmorphics, Rainbow simply said with his mind *"FIRE"*, and six hundred dragons did so, obliterating all traces of Weld and the atmorphics to a fine dust. And as the moon came out from the clouds again, everything looked clean and new.

"Well, That's that!" said Blaze, "it all looks as good as new. I'll send a few down to burn up the one on the ground, keep it all tidy, Eh what1 Now I think it's time some young ones met their families, don't you? It's almost dawn; imagine their amazement at seeing an army of dragons of all colours flying to them in formation as the sun rises. I always think we look best in morning light you know! He he."

So, after checking all the fires were out and no-one was hurt the dragons took off, and led by Rainbow and Pearl and flanked by Sabre, Blaze and his warrior dragons, the army of dragons left for Volcano Valley and their lost younglings who were home at last.

And, may I tell you this dear reader, the Dragon Roar was awesome. Even the younglings added their voices and the echo reverberated round Decagon for hours.

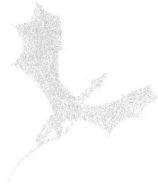

Glossary of the Dragons. (The Goodies)

Rainbow. The leader of the Dragons who represents every dragon colour and can change at will. He is part of the quest searching for his missing partner Pearl.

Pearl. Joint leader with Rainbow who vanished along with a clutch of eggs. She is a powerful white dragon afraid of no-one. How did she get captured?. Why can she not use her telepathy?.

Blaze. A red dragon second in command to Rainbow and Pearl. A warrior dragon, brave, intelligent and ferocious. She is also a telepath and has the power of invisibility and is suspected of having some magical powers including fire.

Meteor. A blue male dragon, also telepathic. A jaunty character but highly reliable. One of Rainbows' cohorts he develops the power of shooting stars and lightning bolts. Favourite phrases are "Dragon plop" and "Bring it on".

Aura. The gold dragon, her special powers is transmutation of metals and shape shifting. She becomes a telepath during the quest. One of the defender guardians she can also do magic.

Green - Peridot. A little green dragon who grows into Peridot. Previous prisoner of the ogres who develops the power of growth and healing as well as telepathy. She is a formidable scrapper and a fierce friend.

Topaz. A pale purple dragon, she is a gentle motherly dragon but will fight to the death as a defender if needed. She has the power to smell out good and evil and can use her non-fire breath to calm beings down and even send them to sleep. A telepath, her fire breath is an intense white heat.

Misty. A deep purple dragon, teacher and a warrior. Her power is music and song, like the sirens of legend. It is thought she is a Sea Dragon and can use her voice like hypnosis. She has been seen to turn rocks and land into water and lava into land.

Rae. A silver and light blue dragon. A warrior dragon who has the power of using dragon fire as fire bolts and quills like arrows from her tail. She too is a telepath.

Emerald. A bronze dragon, she is a teacher and defender of the younglings. Her power is communication with all living things. She is capable of breathing fire at least a hundred metres, maybe more. Also a telepath.

Nattie. A pretty pink dragon. Held prisoner in the walled garden. She is a happiness dragon. She has also made friends with two of the castle's ghosts who cause mischief all over the place and cannot be caught.

THE DRAGONS OF DECAGON

Skye. A blue dragon from the adopted colony, He has become a worthy warrior and is best friends with Meteor.

Sabre. Is Rainbows' twin but he is black. He is the Lord of the Sea Dragons and only changes colour in water. His power is dominance of the seas and manipulation of the water and waves. An intelligent and formidable warrior, he and Rainbow can interchange dominions at times.

Coral. Sabres' mate, she is a healer and warrior. She works with the Merpeople and educates the younglings. Like Pearl she is gentle with a will of iron.

Pulsar. Skye's' father, rescued from certain death by Misty and her team. Joins with the Decagon colony and quite happily accepts Rainbow as leader.

Astral. A terracotta coloured dragon who is a warrior guardian who will protect the younglings. She will fight to the death.

Bowlder. Topaz's mate who is a silver warrior.

Cloud. The mate of Comet and mother of Skye and Star.

Argon. Sea dragon team leader appointed Misty's bodyguard.

Ice. A bluish and white dragon who was lost with her brother Squib when their eggs were ditched by Weld. They are Pearl and Rainbows' younglings.

Shadow and Gravel. Older Keepers and warriors looking after volcano camp and keeping the fires burning.

<u>Sol.</u> A large gold dragon, a new warrior but very smart.

<u>Rock.</u> A grey dragon, unhappy with his colour till it makes him ideal as a scout on the rocky pinnacles and in the castle.

<u>Spike.</u> The discovery that he can become invisible leads the search for more "gifted" younglings.

<u>Beech and Elm.</u> Heroic ghosts of tree sprites aiding the dragons and causing mischief.

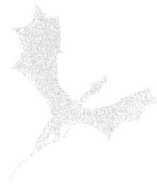

Glossary Of The Not So Good Ones

Weld. Ogre of the black castle who plots to steal the dragon's power.

Goblins. Used by Weld to steal dragon eggs and other nasty things. The masters of Green before her rescue.

Grawks. Nasty big birdlike creatures, a cross between a gryphon and a large hawk. Not very clever they obey every order given by the ogres.

Wolfcrabs. Large crabs with a scaly wolf-like head and wicked teeth that would rip you apart. Able to travel on land as well as in water it was good to avoid their claws which could pull you apart.

Atmorphics. They are the size of a whale, a cross between a shark and a giant squid which propelled itself through the air with its tentacles which could weave patterns and emit hypnotic colours.

Norgra. The usurper of Comets dragons who along with his cronies have gold fever.

www.ingramcontent.com/pod-product-compliance
Lightning Source LLC
Chambersburg PA
CBHW050732030426
42336CB00012B/1525